Pass the Florida Pharmacy Law Exam: A Study Guide and Review for the MPJE

by Sarah Fichuk, Pharm.D., BCPS

Although the author and publisher have made every effort to ensure that the information in this book was correct at press time, the author and publisher do not assume and hereby disclaim any liability to any party for any loss, damage, or disruption caused by errors or omissions, whether such errors or omissions result from negligence, accident, or any other cause.

This book is not intended as a substitute for the legal advice. The reader should consult a competent professional.

NAPLEX®, MPJE®, and NABP® are federally registered trademarks owned by the National Association of Boards of Pharmacy (NABP®). This book is in no way endorsed, sponsored, or authorized by NABP®.
Copyright © 2013 by Sarah E. Fichuk
All rights reserved. This book or any portion thereof
may not be reproduced or used in any manner whatsoever
without the express written permission of the publisher
except for the use of brief quotations in a book review.
Printed in the United States of America
First Printing, 2013
Straight A's Publishing
www.StraightAsPublishing.com

Table of Contents

Table of Contents 5
Section One: Introduction 15
Test Overview 15
    Federal Laws and Rules Tested on the MPJE® 15
    When to Schedule Your Exams 16
    Actually Taking the Test 17
    Warning/Disclaimer 17
    The "Golden Rule" for Pharmacy Law 20
    Acronyms 21
Section Two: Federal Laws and Rules 23
    Federal Food, Drug, and Cosmetic Act 23
    Adultered 24
    Misbranded 24
OTC Label Requirements 25
    Other OTC Rules 25
    Recalls 25
    Advertising 26
    Pregnancy Categories 26
    Plan B Rules 27
Section Three: Federal Controlled Substance Laws 29
    Schedule I Controlled Substances 29
    Schedule II Controlled Substances 29
    Schedule III Controlled Substances 30
    Schedule IV Controlled Substances 30
    Schedule V Controlled Substances 31
    DEA Facts 31
    DEA Registration 31
    Prescriptions 31
    Prescription Requirements 32
    DEA Registration Numbers 33
    Partial Refills of Schedule III, IV, and V 33
    Refill Authorizations for Schedule III, IV, and V 33

Data Processing and Storage Requirements 34
DEA Form 222 34
Completing a DEA Form 222 34
Who May Sign a DEA Form 222? 35
Ordering Drugs Using DEA Form 222 35
Emergency Schedule II Prescriptions 35
Transfer of Business 36
Disposing of Controlled Substances by a Reverse
Distributor 37
Disposing of Controlled Substances at a Pharmacy 37
Returning a Controlled Substance Prescription 37
Theft or Significant Loss 38
Inventory Requirements 38
Authorized Agent of the Prescriber 38
Electronic Prescribing of Controlled Substances 39
Central Filling of Controlled Substances 39
Prescribing Methadone for Pain 40
Detoxification or Maintenance Treatment 40
Transferring Controlled Substance Prescriptions 41
Section Four: Compounding Sterile Preparations 45
Personnel 45
Pharmacists 47
Pharmacy Technicians and Pharmacy Technician
Trainees 47
Documentation of Training 47
Operational Standards 48
Other Rules 48
Microbial Contamination Risk Levels 49
   Low-risk level compounded sterile preparations 49

   Low-Risk Level compounded sterile preparations with 12-hour or fewer beyond-use date 50

   Medium-risk level compounded sterile preparations 50

   High-risk level compounded sterile preparations 51

   Immediate Use Compounded Sterile Preparations 53

6

- Environment 54
- Cytotoxic Drugs 55
- Cleaning and Disinfecting the Sterile Compounding Areas 55
- Personnel Cleansing and Garbing 56
- Section Five: Pseudoephederine Laws 59
- Federal 59
- Section Six: Florida Comprehensive Drug Abuse Prevention and Control Act 61
  - Definitions 61
  - Standards and Schedules 64
  - Scheduling Controlled Substances 66
  - Controlled Substance Prescriptions 66
  - Out of State Controlled Substance Prescriptions 67
  - Controlled Substance Prescriptions 67
  - Controlled Substance Prescription Requirements 67
  - Controlled Substance Prescription Label Requirements 68
  - Schedule II Prescriptions 68
  - Controlled Substance Prescriptions 68
  - Dispensing by a Practitioner 69
  - Prescription Labeling 70
  - Treatment Programs for Impaired Practitioners 70
  - Written Prescriptions for Medicinal Drugs 77
  - Controlled Substance Prescribing for the Treatment of Chronic Nonmalignant Pain 77
- Section Seven: Florida Law Chapter 465 - Pharmacy 83
  - Definitions 83
  - Sterile Compounding Definitions 87
  - Board of Pharmacy 94
  - Licensure by Examination 94
  - Licensure by Endorsement 95
  - Renewal of License 96
  - Continuing Professional Pharmaceutical Education 96
  - Reactivation of License 96

Consultant Pharmacist License 96
Ordering and Evaluating Laboratory or Clinical Testing
.... 97
Nuclear Pharmacists... 97
Pharmacy Interns.. 98
Pharmacy Technicians 98
Violations and Penalties 100
Registration of Nonresident Pharmacies 102
Disciplinary Actions 104
Authority to Inspect... 108
Community Pharmacies; Permits 109
Institutional Pharmacies; Permits 110
Nuclear Pharmacy Permits 113
Special Pharmacy Permits.. 113
Internet Pharmacy Permits 113
Pharmacies; General Requirements 115
Pharmacy Permittee; Disciplinary Action 116
Automated Pharmacy Systems Used By Long-term Care
Facilities, Hospices, or State Correctional Institutions 118
Promoting Sale of Certain Drugs Prohibited 119
Substitution of Drugs... 119
Expiration Date of Medicinal Drugs; Display; Related Use
and Storage Instructions 120
Filling of Certain Prescriptions 120
Centralized Prescription Filling.. 122
Common Database 123
Emergency Prescription Refill 123
Dispensing Practitioner.. 123
Dispensing of Medicinal Drugs Pursuant to Facsimile of
Prescription 126
Rebates Prohibited 127
Pharmacist's Order for Medicinal Drugs........................ 127
Medicaid Audits of Pharmacies... 129
Administration of Influenza Virus Immunizations 131
Section Eight: Florida Law Chapter 64B16-25...................133

8

Probable Cause Panel 133
Initial License Fees 133
Active License Renewal Fees 133
Inactive License Election 134
Retired License Election 134
Delinquent License Reversion 134
CE for Pharmacist 135
CE for a Consultant Pharmacist 136
CE for a Nuclear Pharmacist 136
CE for a Registered Pharmacy Technician 137
Influenza Immunization Certification Program 137
Exemptions for Members of the Armed Forces; Spouses
.... 137
Examination Requirement 138
Licensure by Examination; Application 138
Licensure by Examination; Foreign Pharmacy Graduates
.... 138
Pharmacy Intern Registration Internship Requirements (U.S. Pharmacy Students/Graduates) 139
Pharmacy Intern Registration and Internship Requirements (Foreign Pharmacy Graduates) 140
Licensure by Endorsement 142
Consultant Pharmacist Licensure 143
Nuclear Pharmacist Licensure 144
CE for Nuclear Pharmacist License Renewal 146
Subject Matter for Continuing Education to Order and Evaluate Laboratory Tests 146
Requirements for Pharmacy Technician Registration 147
Standards for Approval of Registered Pharmacy Technician Training Programs 148
Pharmacy Interns; Registration; Employment 149
Tripartite Continuing Education Committee 150
Continuing Education Records Requirements 150
Section Nine: Pharmacy Practice 151

Display of Current License; Pharmacist, Registered, Intern, and Registered Pharmacy Technician Identification 151
Practice of Pharmacy... 151
Oral Prescriptions and Copies 153
Conduct Governing Pharmacists and Pharmacy Permittees 154
Transfer of Prescriptions 155
Ordering and Evaluation of Laboratory Tests 155
General Terms and Conditions to Be Followed by a Pharmacist When Ordering and Dispensing Approved Medicinal Drug Products 155
Prescription Refills 157
Medicinal Drugs Which May Be Ordered by Pharmacists 157
Fluoride Containing Products That May Be Ordered by Pharmacists.. 161
Standards of Practice - Continuous Quality Improvement Program 161
Registered Pharmacy Technician, to Pharmacist Ratio 161
Registered Pharmacy Technician Responsibilities 161
Responsibilities of the Pharmacist................................... 163
Policies and Procedures 163
Negative Drug Formulary 163
Identification of Manufacturer 164
Positive Drug Formulary 165
Duty of Pharmacist to Inform Regarding Drug Substitution 165
Possession and Disposition of Sample Medicinal Drugs 165
Definition of Compounding 166
Standards of Practice for Compounding Sterile Preparations (CSPs).. 168
Requirement for Patient Records 174

Prospective Drug Use Review 175
Patient Counseling 175
Standards of Practice - Drug Therapy Management 175
Standards of Practice for the Dispensing of Controlled
Substances for Treatment of Pain 177
Prescription Area Accessible to Inspection 178
Sink and Running Water, Sufficient Space, Refrigeration,
Sanitation, Equipment 178
Patient Consultation Area 179
All Permits – Labels and Labeling of Medicinal Drugs. 179
Regulation of Daily Operating Hours 183
Prescription Department; Padlock; Sign: "Prescription
Department Closed." 184
Outdated Pharmaceuticals 184
Unit Dose and Customized Patient Medication Package
Returns by In-patients 185
Unclaimed Prescriptions 185
All Permits – Storage of Legend Drugs; Prepackaging. 186
Record Maintenance Systems for Community, Special-
Limited Community, Special-Closed Systems, Special-
Parenteral/Enteral, and Nuclear Permits 187
Requirements for an Automated Pharmacy System in a
Community Pharmacy 190
Closing of a Pharmacy; Transfer of Prescription Files 194
Change of Ownership 195
Transfer of Medicinal Drugs; Change of Ownership;
Closing of a Pharmacy 196
Destruction of Controlled Substances – Institutional
Pharmacies 197
Destruction of Controlled Substances All Permittees
(excluding Nursing Homes) 197
Centralized Prescription Filling, Delivering and
Returning 198
Pharmacy Common Database 202

Institutional Permit – Consultant Pharmacist of Record 204
Class I Institutional Permit and Class II Institutional Permit – Labels and Labeling of Medicinal Drugs for Inpatients of a Nursing Home 205
Transmission of Starter Dose Prescriptions for Patients in Class I Institutional or Modified II B Facilities 206
Institutional Class II Dispensing 208
Institutional Class II Pharmacy – Emergency Department Dispensing 209
Class II Institutional Pharmacy Department Security . 210
Class II Institutional Pharmacies – Automated Distribution and Packaging 210
Remote Medication Order Processing for Class II Institutional Pharmacies 215
Automated Pharmacy System – Long Term Care, Hospice, and Prison 218
Modified Class II Institutional Pharmacies 223
Special Pharmacies 228
Special Pharmacy – Limited Community Permit 229
Sterile Products and Special Parenteral/Enteral Compounding 229
Special – Closed System Pharmacy 235
Special – Non Resident (Mail Service) 236
Special Pharmacy – ESRD 236
Special Pharmacy – Parenteral/Enteral Extended Scope Permit 239
Special-ALF 242
Definitions – Nuclear Pharmacy 243
Nuclear Pharmacy – General Requirements 244
Nuclear Pharmacy – Minimum Requirements 246
Animal Control Shelter Permits 246
Section Ten: Review and Practice Questions 249
Things You Should Probably Know 249
Review Questions 265

Section One: Introduction

Test Overview
- Online registration at www.nabp.net
- Computer-based test
- Adaptive technology selects the next question based on the answers to your previous questions
- No distinction between federal and state law (answer according to the strictest rule)
- 2 hours for 90 questions
- 75 scored questions
- 15 pretest questions
- Scored questions are not identified
- Minimum passing score is 75 in a range of 0–100
- Scaled score (compares your score to the minimum acceptable score)
- Cannot change an answer once it has been confirmed
- Cannot go back and review questions
- All questions must be answered in order
- Cannot skip questions
- Scores are available online at www.nabp.net within 7 business days (usually in 2-3 business days)

Federal Laws and Rules Tested on the MPJE®
- Federal Food, Drug and Cosmetic Act
- Federal Controlled Substance Act
- Poison Prevention Packaging Act
- Pseudoephedrine Laws

How to Use This Book

This book is a compilation of most of the Florida laws and rules pertaining to pharmacy. Many of the laws and rules have been edited down to be more concise. But some of the laws I have left as is because I feel that reading them leads to better understanding. There is also a section at the end which contains a review sheet of commonly tested items along with 35 review questions.

I recommend that you make sure you read the test objectives for the Florida MPJE which are available on their website prior to reading this book. That way you know what information to pay special attention to while studying. Everything is important, but there are certain things you must know.

Particularly focus on all the information in the controlled substances section. Read that section again just prior to taking the test. It would be better to be over-prepared rather than underprepared. This is one of the most important tests of your career.

When to Schedule Your Exams

I recommend focusing on only one exam at time, either the NAPLEX® or the MPJE®. You will probably need a minimum of a week to study for the MPJE®, if not two weeks. So keep that in mind when scheduling your exams.

Actually Taking the Test

There will be answers like "1 and 2," "2 only," and "1, 2 and 3."

Read each question carefully. Do not read too much into the question or try to overanalyze—think in straightforward terms and go with your first choice when reading the answers.

Do not rush through each question. You have plenty of time to take the test—over a minute for each question—and some will be easy and straightforward, so don't panic about time. Some questions, you have to guess at, so don't get discouraged.

Warning/Disclaimer

This book is not intended to be comprehensive review of all pharmacy law. Many of the rules and laws applicable to the practice of pharmacy were **NOT** included because the author felt they were unlikely to be on the MPJE®. This book is a study guide to help pharmacists and pharmacy students pass the federal law questions on the MPJE®. It is intended to be a supplement to the law class taken in pharmacy school.

If the reader has concerns over a statement made in this book or has further questions, the reader should read the actual law referenced.

A word of caution: Even if you have worked retail as a technician for years, you still need to study to pass this test. The pharmacy you worked at may not have been following the law as written.

Test Objectives

Federal and State Controlled Substance Acts and Regulations
- Definitions of controlled substances
- Who registers with DEA and DPS and how
- Storage requirements for controlled substances
- What records must be maintained
- Central record keeping requirements and restrictions
- Obtaining, executing, and storing DEA order forms
- Returning controlled substances to supplier
- Disposing expired or contaminated controlled substances
- Prescription requirements for Schedule II–V
- Refill requirements for Schedule II–V
- Emergency refill requirements for Schedule III–V
- Partial dispensing of Schedule II and Schedule III–V
- Emergency oral order of Schedule II
- Federal "transfer warning" statement
- OTC sale of Schedule V products
- Schedule II prescription requirements and exceptions
- Criteria to place a drug in the five schedules
- Recognizing commonly used controlled substances and their schedules
- Reporting theft/loss to DEA and DPS
- Employee screening
- Procedures for closing a business
- Legal use of methadone
- Methadone to treat addiction
- Using Subutex® or Suboxone®
- Physicians' designated agents
- Faxed Schedule II prescriptions

Federal and State Food, Drug, and Cosmetic Acts
- Definitions
- Adultered
- Misbranded
- Registration requirements for manufacturers and distributors
- Illegal pharmacist acts under the Durham-Humphrey Amendments
- Requirements for manufacturers' labels
- How long to keep prescriptions
- Recall classification system
- Good Manufacturing Practice

Miscellaneous
- Exceptions to child-resistant packaging
- Mailing controlled substances

The "Golden Rule" for Pharmacy Law

You are required to follow the strictest standard when comparing federal and state law. For example federal law allows 3 different filing systems for prescriptions but Texas only allows 1. Therefore the correct standard to follow is the Texas law.

Also keep all records for a minimum of 2 years.

Acronyms

ACPE – Accreditation Council for Pharmacy Education
ACLS – Advanced Cardiac Life Support
BCLS – Basic Cardiac Life Support
CE – Continuing education
DEA – Drug Enforcement Administration
DPS – Department of Public Safety
FDA – Food and Drug Administration
FPGEC – Foreign Pharmacy Graduate Equivalency Commission
FPGEE – Foreign Pharmacy Graduate Equivalency Examination
GED – General education development
HEPA – High efficiency particulate air
HIPAA – Health Insurance Portability and Accountability Act
IPA – Isopropyl alcohol
ISO – International Organization of Standardization
MPJE – Multistate Pharmacy Jurisprudence Examination
MSA – Metropolitan statistical area
NABP – National Association of Boards of Pharmacy
NAPLEX – North American Pharmacy Licensing Examination
NDC – National drug code
OTC – Over the counter
PALS – Pediatric Advanced Life Support
PIC – Pharmacist-in-charge
PMR – Patient medication record
PTCB – Pharmacy Technician Certification Board
SOP – Standard operating procedure
SWFI – Sterile water for injection
TPN – Total parentral nutrition
USP/NF – United States Pharmacopeia/National Formulary

Section Two: Federal Laws and Rules

Federal Food, Drug, and Cosmetic Act
Purpose: protect the public health by requiring safe, effective, and properly labeled drugs and devices

History
- **1906 Pure Food and Drug Act**
  - Purity standards only; no efficacy requirements
- **1938 Federal Food, Drug, and Cosmetic Act**
  - Safety standards only; no efficacy requirements
- **1951 Durham-Humphrey Amendments**
  - Created OTC and prescription drug categories
- **1962 Kefauver-Harris Amendment**
  - Efficacy requirements
- **1976 Medical Device Amendment**
  - Added regulatory authority over devices
- **1983 Orphan Drug Act**
  - Incentives to create drugs for rare diseases (longer patent life)
- **1984 Drug Price Competition and Patent Restoration Act**
  - Patent holders received 5 years of patent life because of the FDA's process to review drug applications
- **1988 Prescription Drug Marketing Act of 1987**
  - State licensing of wholesale distributors
  - Banned reimportation of prescription drugs
  - Banned sale, trade, or purchase of drug samples
- **1997 FDA Modernization Act**
  - Requires "Rx only" on the prescription legend
- **1999 Over-the-Counter Labeling Requirements**
  - Standardized OTC labeling

Adultered
Refers to the actual makeup or composition of the drug
- Containing any filthy substance
- May have been contaminated in preparation/storage/packaging
- Good manufacturing practices not followed
- Container may contaminate the drug
- Unsafe color additive
- Strength differs from what listed on the label (A 5% difference is okay)
- Misfilled: drug has been substituted

Misbranded
Refers to the drug labeling
- Labeling is false or misleading
- Manufacturer's labeling requirements:
    - Name and address of manufacturer
    - Quantity
    - Generic and brand name of the drug (if applicable)
    - Strength of the drug
    - Information for use
    - Warnings against use
    - Expiration date
- Pharmacist filling a prescription without authorization from prescriber
- Counterfeit drug
- Packaging violates Poison Prevention Packaging Act
- Packaging not containing all the words or statements as required by law

OTC Label Requirements
- Must contain adequate *directions* for use—in comparison, prescription drug labeling must contain adequate *information* for use
- Display panel with name of product
- Name and address of manufacturer/packer/distributor
- Quantity in container
- Cautions and warnings
- Adequate directions for safe and effective use (must be written for a layperson)
- "Drug Facts" must contain
    - Active ingredients
    - Purpose
    - Uses – indications
    - Warnings
    - Directions
    - Other information
    - Inactive ingredients
    - Questions? (optional) followed by telephone number

Other OTC Rules
- Prescribed an OTC but dose is higher than OTC limits: must be written and filled as a prescription
- If an OTC is written as a prescription, then it needs to be filled as a prescription, but a pharmacist can sell an OTC if he or she feels it to be in the best interest of the patient

Recalls
- FDA has no authority to recall drugs, only devices
- **Class I recall** – reasonable probability exposure will cause serious adverse health effects or death

- **Class II recall** – may cause temporary or medically reversible adverse health effects
- **Class III recall** – not likely to cause adverse health effects

Advertising
- Prescription drug advertising – regulated by FDA
- OTC advertising – regulated by Federal Trade Commission
- Pharmacists may advertise
    - Provide pricing information—must include brand/generic name, strength, dosage form, and price charged for a specific quantity
    - Availability of professional services
    - Price stated must include all charges to consumer; mailing and delivery fees may be stated separately

Pregnancy Categories

Category A
Adequate and well-controlled studies have failed to demonstrate a risk to the fetus in the first trimester of pregnancy (and there is no evidence of risk in later trimesters).

Category B
Animal reproduction studies have failed to demonstrate a risk to the fetus, and there are no adequate and well-controlled studies in pregnant women.

Category C
Animal reproduction studies have shown an adverse effect on the fetus, and there are no adequate and well-controlled studies in humans, but potential benefits may warrant use of the drug in pregnant women despite potential risks.

Category D
There is positive evidence of human fetal risk based on adverse reaction data from investigational or marketing experience or studies in humans, but potential benefits may warrant use of the drug in pregnant women despite potential risks.

Category X
Studies in animals or humans have demonstrated fetal abnormalities and/or there is positive evidence of human fetal risk based on adverse reaction data from investigational or marketing experience, and the risks involved in use of the drug in pregnant women clearly outweigh potential benefits.

Plan B Rules

- Plan B, Plan B One-Step, and their generic versions are allowed to be sold over-the-counter to consumers 17 years and older and available by prescription only for women 16 years and younger
- Only sold in pharmacies/stores staffed by a licensed pharmacist
- Will be kept behind the pharmacy counter because the packaging has both over-the-counter and prescription labeling
- Proof of age via personal identification will be required at time of purchase
- Men may purchase Plan B—the wording is "to consumers 17 years and older"

Section Three: Federal Controlled Substance Laws

Schedule I Controlled Substances
- High potential for abuse
- No currently accepted medical use
- Lack of accepted safety for use under medical supervision
- Examples:
    - Heroin
    - Lysergic acid diethylamide (LSD)
    - Marijuana (cannabis)
    - Peyote
    - 3,4-methylenedioxymethamphetamine ("ecstasy")
- ** Use of peyote by the Native American Church is allowed, but manufacturers and distributors of peyote must be registered

Schedule II Controlled Substances
- High potential for abuse which may lead to severe psychological or physical dependence
- Examples:
    - Narcotics
        - Hydromorphone (Dilaudid®)
        - Methadone (Dolophine®)
        - Meperidine (Demerol®)
        - Oxycodone (OxyContin®)
        - Fentanyl (Sublimaze® or Duragesic®)
    - Stimulants
        - Amphetamine (Dexedrine®, Adderall®)
        - Methamphetamine (Desoxyn®)
        - Methylphenidate (Ritalin®)
    - Others

- Cocaine
- Amobarbital
- Glutethimide
- Pentobarbital

Schedule III Controlled Substances

- Potential for abuse less than substances in schedules I or II and abuse may lead to moderate or low physical dependence or high psychological dependence
- Examples:
  - Narcotics
    - Combination products containing less than 15 milligrams of hydrocodone per dosage unit (Vicodin®)
    - Products containing not more than 90 milligrams of codeine per dosage unit (Tylenol with codeine®)
  - Products to treat opioid addiction
    - Buprenorphine (Suboxone® and Subutex®)
  - Others
    - Benzphetamine (Didrex®)
    - Phendimetrazine
    - Ketamine
    - Anabolic steroids

Schedule IV Controlled Substances

- Low potential for abuse relative to substances in Schedule III
- Effective 1/11/12: carisoprodol will be Schedule IV
- Examples:
  - Alprazolam (Xanax®)
  - Clonazepam (Klonopin®)
  - Clorazepate (Tranxene®)
  - Diazepam (Valium®)

- Lorazepam (Ativan®)
- Midazolam (Versed®)
- Temazepam (Restoril®)
- Triazolam (Halcion®)

Schedule V Controlled Substances
- Low potential for abuse relative to substances listed in schedule IV
- Contain limited quantities of certain narcotics
- Generally used for antitussive, antidiarrheal, and analgesic purposes
- Examples
    - Cough preparations containing not more than 200 milligrams of codeine per 100 milliliters or per 100 grams (Robitussin AC® and Phenergan with Codeine®)

DEA Facts
- The U.S. Drug Enforcement Administration (DEA) is a component of the U.S. Department of Justice
- "responsible for enforcing the controlled substances laws and regulations of the United States"

DEA Registration
- All DEA registrants: register every 3 years with DEA form 224 (for pharmacies)
- DEA sends out renewal form 60 days prior to expiration date
- Must notify DEA in writing if have not received renewal form 45 days prior to expiration date

Prescriptions
- Must be for legitimate medical purposes

- Practitioner must be acting in the usual course of their professional practice
- Pharmacists also have a corresponding responsibility with the practitioner for the proper prescribing and dispensing
- Writing a prescription "for office use" is not allowed; practitioner must order directly from a supplier or distributor
- Narcotic prescriptions may not be written for "detoxification treatment" or "maintenance treatment"
- Physicians should not write prescriptions for themselves or family members (but no law against it)
- Practitioners do not need to register with the DEA if they work at a hospital/institution (can use the hospital's DEA number and then the code assigned to them)
- Schedule III–V are allowed 5 refills in the 6 months from the date written

Prescription Requirements
- A prescription must be written in ink or indelible pencil or typewritten and must be manually signed by the practitioner
- A prescription for a controlled substance must include the following information:
    - Date of issue
    - Patient's name and address
    - Practitioner's name, address, and DEA registration number
    - Drug name
    - Drug strength
    - Dosage form
    - Quantity prescribed
    - Directions for use
    - Number of refills (if any) authorized; and

- Manual signature of prescriber

DEA Registration Numbers
There is an easy formula to determine if a DEA number is valid
- Add the 1st, 3rd, and 5th digits of the DEA number
- Add the 2nd, 4th and 6th digits and multiply by 2
- Add the results of those two calculations
- The last digit from the sum of the first two steps should be the same as the 7th digit in the DEA number
- Example: BF1234563
  - $1 + 3 + 5 = 9$
  - $2 + 4 + 6 = 12 \times 2 = 24$
  - $9 + 24 = 33$
  - So the 7th digit should be "3"
  - Therefore this DEA number is valid

Partial Refills of Schedule III, IV, and V
Partial refills are allowed, provided that each partial filling is dispensed and recorded in the same manner as a refilling (e.g., date refilled, amount dispensed, initials of dispensing pharmacist), the total quantity dispensed in all partial fillings does not exceed the total quantity prescribed, and no dispensing occurs after 6 months past the date of issue.

Refill Authorizations for Schedule III, IV, and V
- Prescriber allowed to orally authorize additional refills
- Not allowed to exceed 5 refills in a 6-month time period from the date the prescription was originally written
- Quantity of each additional refill must be the same as or less than the initial quantity authorized
- New and separate prescription required for any additional quantities above and beyond the "5 refills in 6 months" limit

Data Processing and Storage Requirements
- Pharmacists are allowed to store refill information in a computer
- System must produce a daily hard copy readout of all processed controlled substance refills
- Each individual pharmacist must verify the information is correct and date and sign the hard copy readout
- A logbook may be used instead of the daily hard copy readout, where each pharmacist must sign a statement every day that says the information entered into the computer that day was correct

DEA Form 222
- Required for the sale or transfer of Schedule I or II controlled substances
- Pharmacies may transfer controlled substances to other pharmacies as long as the total amount is up to 5% of the total amount of controlled substances dispensed in a year without having to register as a wholesaler
- Carbon triplicate: Copy 1, Copy 2, and Copy 3
- Each form is numbered serially
- Preprinted with name, address, and registration number of the registrant; the authorized activity; and the schedules of the registrant
  - Cannot be changed
  - In case of changed information, must have new forms made

Completing a DEA Form 222
- Must be completed in ink, indelible pencil, or typewritten
- Only one item per numbered line on the form
  - "One item" means one drug, strength, and package size

- The number of lines completed must be filled in at the bottom of the form
- Name and address of the supplier must be filled in

Who May Sign a DEA Form 222?
- Individual who signed the DEA registration
- Individual who is authorized through the execution of a power of attorney by an individual who signed the DEA registration

Ordering Drugs Using DEA Form 222
- Purchaser fills out the form and submits Copy 1 and 2 to the supplier and keeps Copy 3 for their records
- Supplier fills the order and records on Copy 1 and 2 the number of commercial or bulk containers supplied on each item and the date shipped to purchaser
- Order may be filled in part, with the balance shipped within 60 days of the date on the form
- After 60 days, the order form is no longer valid
- May only be shipped to the address on the form
- Supplier keeps Copy 1 and forwards Copy 2 to the DEA
- When the purchaser receives the shipment, they must note how many containers received on each item and the date received on Copy 3
- Order form may not be filled if it
    - Is not complete, legible, or properly prepared, executed, or endorsed
    - Shows any adulteration, erasure, or change of any description

Emergency Schedule II Prescriptions
- DEA regulations limit an emergency oral prescription to the quantity necessary to treat the patient during the emergency period

- Oral emergency prescriptions must immediately be reduced to writing by the pharmacist and must contain all the information ordinarily required in a prescription, except for the signature of the prescribing individual practitioner
- If the prescribing individual practitioner is not known to the pharmacist, the pharmacist must make a reasonable effort to determine that the oral authorization came from a registered individual practitioner, which may include a call back to the prescribing individual practitioner and/or other good faith efforts to ensure the practitioner's identity
- An emergency situation is defined as all of the following:
    - Immediate administration of the controlled substance is necessary for proper treatment
    - No appropriate alternative treatments are available including non–Schedule II controlled substances
    - Not reasonably possible for the physician to provide a written prescription prior to dispensing

Transfer of Business
- Notify DEA 14 days prior to transfer
- Day of transfer: complete inventory, which serves as both the closing and opening inventories
- Transferring schedule II – use official DEA 222 order form
- Transferring schedule III–V – separate document with
    - Name of drug
    - Dosage form
    - Strength
    - Quantity
    - Date transferred

- Names, addresses, and DEA numbers of the pharmacies

Disposing of Controlled Substances by a Reverse Distributor
- May send to a reverse distributor registered with the DEA
    - Schedule II – DEA 222
    - Schedule III–V – written record of name, form, strength, quantity
- Reverse distributor will submit to the DEA form 41 when the controlled substances have been destroyed
- Disposal by those **not** registered with the DEA (ex. long-term care facilities)

Disposing of Controlled Substances at a Pharmacy
- Once a year, retail pharmacies may request DEA permission to dispose of controlled substances that are unwanted, expired, etc.
- Pharmacy completes DEA Form 41 that lists all drugs to be destroyed
- Pharmacy sends letter to DEA with the form at least 14 days in advance, asking for permission
    - Letter contains the proposed date of destruction, method of destruction, and identity of the two witnesses (licensed physician, pharmacist, mid-level practitioner, nurse, or state or local law enforcement officer)

Returning a Controlled Substance Prescription
- An individual may not return unused controlled substance prescription medication to the pharmacy

- There are no provisions in federal laws and regulations to acquire controlled substances from a non-registrant (e.g., individual patient)
- An individual may dispose of their own controlled substance medication without approval from DEA

Theft or Significant Loss
- Notify DEA within one business day of the discovery
- Notify local law enforcement and state regulatory agencies
- Complete DEA form 106

Inventory Requirements
- Actual count of Schedule II
- Estimate count of Schedule III, IV, and V if bottle is <1,000 count
- Actual count of Schedule III, IV, and V if bottle >1,000 count
- Keep records for 2 years
- Records and inventories of Schedule I and II must be kept separately from all other records
- Records and inventories of Schedule III, IV, and V must be kept separately from all other records or readily retrievable
- Inventory of all controlled substances must be done every 2 years

Authorized Agent of the Prescriber
- An authorized agent of the prescriber may
    - Prepare a controlled substance prescription for the signature of the prescriber
    - Orally communicated a prescriber's Schedule III–V prescription to a pharmacist
    - Transmit by fax a prescriber's written Schedule II prescription to a pharmacist

- An authorized agent **cannot** orally communicate an emergency Schedule II prescription to a pharmacist
- To be an agent of the prescriber, a detailed written document must be created and specifies the authority being granted
- DEA also recommends providing a copy to pharmacies likely to receive prescriptions from the prescriber's agent
- Pharmacists still retain responsibility to make sure the controlled substance prescription conforms to the appropriate laws and regulations and is for a legitimate medical purpose

Electronic Prescribing of Controlled Substances
- Practitioners may write electronic controlled substance prescriptions
- Pharmacies may receive, dispense, and archive these electronic prescriptions
- Pharmacies must use specific software approved by the DEA, which must be certified by a third party audit

Central Filling of Controlled Substances
- Central fill pharmacies are permitted to fill the initial and refills of Schedule II, III, IV, and V prescriptions
- May be transmitted electronically or via fax from the community pharmacy
- Community pharmacy writes "CENTRAL FILL" on the face of the original prescription and includes name, address and DEA number of the central fill pharmacy
- Central fill pharmacies must place a label to the packaging showing the local pharmacy name and address as well as a unique identifier to show it was filled at the central fill pharmacy

Prescribing Methadone for Pain
- Federal law and regulations do not restrict the prescribing, dispensing, or administering of any schedule II, III, IV, or V narcotic medication, including methadone, for the treatment of pain, if such treatment is deemed medically necessary by a registered practitioner acting in the usual course of professional practice.
- Use of methadone for the maintenance or detoxification of opioid-addicted individuals, in which case the practitioner is required to be registered with the DEA as a Narcotic Treatment Program (NTP)

Detoxification or Maintenance Treatment
- A practitioner may administer or dispense directly (but not prescribe) a narcotic drug listed in any schedule to a narcotic-dependent person for the purpose of maintenance or detoxification treatment if the practitioner meets both of the following conditions:
    - is separately registered with DEA as a narcotic treatment program
    - complies with DEA regulations regarding treatment qualifications, security, records, and unsupervised use of the drugs
- A physician who is not specifically registered to conduct a narcotic treatment program may administer (but not prescribe) narcotic drugs to a person for the purpose of relieving acute withdrawal symptoms when necessary while arrangements are being made for referral for treatment.

- - No more than 1 day's medication may be administered to the person or for the person's use at one time.
    - Such emergency treatment may be carried out for no more than 3 days and may not be renewed or extended.
- Physicians may administer or dispense narcotic drugs in a hospital to maintain or detoxify a person as an incidental adjunct to a medical or surgical treatment of conditions other than addiction or those with intractable pain

Transferring Controlled Substance Prescriptions
- Allowed one time only
    - If pharmacies electronically share a real-time, online database, pharmacies may transfer up to the maximum refills permitted
- Must be communicated directly between two licensed pharmacists
- Transferring pharmacist
    - Voids the prescription
    - Records the name, address, and DEA number of the pharmacy to which it was transferred
    - Records the name of the pharmacist receiving the prescription
    - Records the date of the transfer and name of the pharmacist performing the transfer
- Receiving pharmacist writes
    - "Transfer" on the face of the prescription
    - Date of issuance of original prescription
    - Original number of refills authorized
    - Date of original dispensing
    - Number of valid refills remaining and date(s) and locations of previous refill(s)

- Pharmacy's name, address, DEA number, and prescription number from which the prescription was transferred
- Name of pharmacist who transferred the prescription
- Pharmacy's name, address, DEA number, and prescription number from which the prescription was originally filled

Dispensing Without a Prescription

A controlled substance listed in Schedules II, III, IV, or V which is not a prescription drug as determined under the Federal Food, Drug, and Cosmetic Act, may be dispensed by a pharmacist without a prescription to a purchaser at retail, provided that:

- Only done by a pharmacist and not by a nonpharmacist employee even if under the supervision of a pharmacist (although after the pharmacist has fulfilled his professional and legal responsibilities set forth in this section, the actual cash, credit transaction, or delivery, may be completed by a nonpharmacist)
- Not more than 240 cc. (8 ounces) of any such controlled substance containing opium, nor more than 120 cc. (4 ounces) of any other such controlled substance nor more than 48 dosage units of any such controlled substance containing opium, nor more than 24 dosage units of any other such controlled substance may be dispensed at retail to the same purchaser in any given 48-hour period
- Purchaser is at least 18 years of age
- Pharmacist requires every purchaser of a controlled substance under this section not known to him to furnish suitable identification (including proof of age where appropriate)

- A bound record book for dispensing of controlled substances under this section is maintained by the pharmacist, which book shall contain the name and address of the purchaser, the name and quantity of controlled substance purchased, the date of each purchase, and the name or initials of the pharmacist who dispensed the substance
- A prescription is not required for distribution or dispensing of the substance pursuant to any other Federal, State or local law
- Central fill pharmacies may not dispense controlled substances to a purchaser at retail pursuant to this section.

Section Four: Compounding Sterile Preparations

Personnel

- A pharmacist shall inspect and approve all components, drug preparation containers, closures, labeling, and any other materials involved in the compounding process
- A pharmacist shall review all compounding records for accuracy and conduct checks during and after the compounding process to ensure that errors have not occurred
- A pharmacist shall be accessible at all times to respond to patients' and other health professionals' questions and needs. Such access may be through a telephone or pager which is answered 24 hours a day
- All pharmacy personnel preparing sterile preparations shall receive didactic and experiential training and competency evaluation through
    - Demonstration
    - Testing (written and practical), as outlined by the pharmacist-in-charge and described in the policy and procedure or training manual
- The aseptic technique of each person compounding or responsible for the direct supervision of personnel compounding sterile preparations shall be observed and evaluated as satisfactory through written and practical tests, and media-fill challenge testing, and such evaluation documented
- Although media-fill tests may be incorporated into the experiential portion of a training program, media-fill tests must be conducted at each pharmacy where an individual compounds sterile preparations. No preparation intended for patient use shall be compounded by an individual until the on-site media-fill

tests test indicates that the individual can competently perform aseptic procedures, except that a pharmacist may temporarily compound sterile preparations and supervise pharmacy technicians compounding sterile preparations without media-fill tests provided the pharmacist:
- o Has completed a recognized course in an accredited college of pharmacy or a course sponsored by an ACPE accredited provider that provides 20 hours of instruction and experience in the areas listed in this subparagraph; **and**
- o Completes the on-site media-fill tests within seven (7) days of commencing work at the pharmacy
- Media-fill test procedures for assessing the preparation of specific types of sterile preparations shall be representative of all types of manipulations, products, risk levels, and batch sizes that personnel preparing that type of sterile preparation are likely to encounter
- The pharmacist-in-charge shall ensure continuing competency of pharmacy personnel through in-service education, training, and media-fill tests to supplement initial training. Personnel competency shall be evaluated
  - o During orientation and training prior to the regular performance of those tasks
  - o Whenever the quality assurance program yields an unacceptable result
  - o Whenever unacceptable techniques are observed; **and**
  - o At least on an annual basis for low- and medium-risk level compounding, and every six (6) months for high-risk level compounding

Pharmacists

All pharmacists who compound sterile preparations for administration to patients or supervise pharmacy technicians and pharmacy technician trainees compounding sterile preparations shall complete through a single course, a minimum of 20 hours of instruction and experience. Such training may be obtained through:
- Completion of a structured on-the-job didactic and experiential training program at the pharmacy that provides 20 hours of instruction and experience. Such training may not be transferred to another pharmacy unless the pharmacies are under common ownership and control and use a common training program; **or**
- Completion of a recognized course in an accredited college of pharmacy or a course sponsored by an ACPE accredited provider that provides 20 hours of instruction and experience

Pharmacy Technicians and Pharmacy Technician Trainees

In addition to specific qualifications for registration, all pharmacy technicians and pharmacy technician trainees who compound sterile preparations for administration to patients shall have initial training obtained through completion of a single course, a minimum of 40 hours of instruction

Documentation of Training

The pharmacy shall maintain a record on each person who compounds sterile preparations. The record shall contain, at a minimum, a written record of initial and in-service training, education, and the results of written and practical testing and media-fill testing of pharmacy personnel.

Operational Standards

Sterile preparations may be compounded in licensed pharmacies
- Upon presentation of a practitioner's prescription drug or medication order based on a valid pharmacist/patient/prescriber relationship
- In anticipation of future prescription drug or medication orders based on routine, regularly observed prescribing patterns (see more on this under non-sterile compounding)
- In reasonable quantities for office use by a practitioner and for use by a veterinarian

Any preparation compounded in anticipation of future prescription drug or medication orders shall be labeled
- Name and strength of the compounded preparation **or** list of the active ingredients and strengths
- Facility's lot number
- Beyond-use date
- Quantity or amount in the container
- Appropriate ancillary instructions, such as storage instructions or cautionary statements, including hazardous drug warning labels where appropriate

Other Rules

- Commercially available products – same conditions as non-sterile compounding
- A pharmacy may enter into an agreement to compound and dispense prescription/medication orders for another pharmacy, provided the pharmacy complies with the title relating to Centralized Prescription Dispensing
- Compounding pharmacies/pharmacists may advertise and promote the fact that they provide sterile

prescription compounding services, which may include specific drug preparations and classes of drugs
- A pharmacy may not compound veterinary preparations for use in food-producing animals except in accordance with federal guidelines

Microbial Contamination Risk Levels
Risk Levels for sterile compounded preparations shall be as outlined in Chapter 797, Pharmacy Compounding—Sterile Preparations of the USP/NF and as listed below

Low-risk level compounded sterile preparations
- The compounded sterile preparations are compounded with aseptic manipulations entirely within ISO Class 5 or better air quality using only sterile ingredients, products, components, and devices
- The compounding involves only transfer, measuring, and mixing manipulations with closed or sealed packaging systems that are preformed promptly and attentively
- Manipulations are limited to aseptically opening ampules, penetrating sterile stoppers on vials with sterile needles and syringes, and transferring sterile liquids in sterile syringes to sterile administration devices and packages of other sterile products
- For a low-risk preparation, the storage periods may not exceed the following periods before administration:
    - 48 hours at controlled room temperature
    - 14 days if stored at a cold temperature
    - 45 days if stored in a frozen state, at minus 20 degrees Celsius or colder
    - For delayed activation device systems, the storage period begins when the device is activated

Examples of Low-Risk Compounding

- Single volume transfers of sterile dosage forms from ampules, bottles, bags, and vials; using sterile syringes with sterile needles, other administration devices, and other sterile containers
- Manually measuring and mixing no more than *three (3)* manufactured products to compound drug admixtures

Low-Risk Level compounded sterile preparations with 12-hour or fewer beyond-use date

- The compounded sterile preparations are compounded in compounding aseptic isolator or compounding aseptic containment isolator that is not ISO Class 5 or better or the compounded sterile preparations are compounded in laminar airflow workbench or a biological safety cabinet that cannot be located within an ISO Class 7 buffer area
- Administration of such compounded sterile preparations must commence within 12 hours of preparation or as recommended in the manufacturers' package insert, whichever is less

Medium-risk level compounded sterile preparations

Medium-risk level compounded sterile preparations are those compounded aseptically under low-risk conditions, and one or more of the following conditions exist

- Multiple individual or small doses of sterile products are combined or pooled to prepare a compounded sterile preparation that will be administered either to multiple patients or to one patient on multiple occasions
- The compounding process includes complex aseptic manipulations other than the single-volume transfer
- The compounding process requires unusually long duration, such as that required to complete the dissolution or homogenous mixing (e.g., reconstitution

of intravenous immunoglobulin or other intravenous protein products)
- The compounded sterile preparations do not contain broad-spectrum bacteriostatic substances and they are administered over several days (e.g., an externally worn infusion device)
- For a medium-risk preparation, the beyond-use dates may not exceed the following time periods before administration:
  - 30 hours at controlled room temperature
  - 9 days at a cold temperature
  - 45 days in solid frozen state, at minus 20 degrees Celsius or colder

Examples of medium-risk compounding
- Compounding of total parenteral nutrition fluids using a manual or automated device, during which there are multiple injections, detachments, and attachments of nutrient-source products to the device or machine to deliver all nutritional components to a final sterile container
- Filling of reservoirs of injection and infusion devices with multiple sterile drug products, and evacuating air from those reservoirs before the filled device is dispensed
- Filling of reservoirs of injection and infusion devices with volumes of sterile drug solutions that will be administered over several days at ambient temperatures between 25 and 40 degrees Celsius (77 and 104 degrees Fahrenheit)
- Transferring volumes from multiple ampules or vials into a single, final sterile container or product

High-risk level compounded sterile preparations
High-risk level compounded sterile preparations are those compounded under any of the following conditions

- Non-sterile ingredients, including manufactured products, are incorporated; or a non-sterile device is employed before terminal sterilization
- Sterile ingredients, components, devices, and mixtures are exposed to air quality inferior to ISO Class 5.
    - This includes storage in environments inferior to ISO Class 5 of opened or partially used packages of manufactured sterile products that lack antimicrobial preservatives
- Non-sterile preparations are exposed no more than 6 hours before being sterilized
- For a high-risk preparation, the beyond-use dates may not exceed the following time periods before administration:
    - 24 hours at controlled room temperature
    - 3 days at a cold temperature
    - 45 days in solid frozen state, at minus 20 degrees or colder
- All high-risk compounded sterile aqueous solutions subjected to terminal sterilization are passed through a filter with a nominal porosity not larger than 1.2 micron preceding or during filling into their final containers to remove particulate matter. Sterilization of high-risk level compounded sterile preparations by filtration shall be performed entirely within an ISO Class 5 or superior air quality environment

Examples of high-risk compounding
- Dissolving non-sterile bulk drug powders to make solutions, which will be terminally sterilized
- Exposing the sterile ingredients and components used to prepare and package compounded sterile preparations to room air quality worse than ISO Class 5
- Measuring and mixing sterile ingredients in non-sterile devices before sterilization is performed

- Assuming, without appropriate evidence or direct determination, that packages of bulk ingredients contain at least 95% by weight of their active chemical moiety and have not been contaminated or adulterated between uses

Immediate Use Compounded Sterile Preparations
For the purpose of emergency or immediate patient care, such situations may include cardiopulmonary resuscitation, emergency room treatment, preparation of diagnostic agents, or critical therapy where the preparation of the compounded sterile preparation under low-risk level conditions would subject the patient to additional risk due to delays in therapy. Compounded sterile preparations are exempted from the requirements described in this paragraph for low-risk, medium-risk, and high-risk level compounded sterile preparations when all of the following criteria are met.
- Only simple aseptic measuring and transfer manipulations are performed with not more than three (3) sterile non-hazardous commercial drug and diagnostic radiopharmaceutical drug products, including an infusion or diluent solution
- Unless required for the preparation, the preparation procedure occurs continuously without delays or interruptions and does not exceed 1 hour
- Administration begins not later than one (1) hour following the completion of preparing the compounded sterile preparation
- When the compounded sterile preparations is not administered by the person who prepared it or its administration is not witnessed by the person who prepared it, the compounded sterile preparation shall bear a label listing patient identification information such as name and identification number(s), the names and amounts of all ingredients, the name or initials of

the person who prepared the compounded sterile preparation, and the exact 1-hour beyond-use time and date
- If administration has not begun within one (1) hour following the completion of preparing the compounded sterile preparation, the compounded sterile preparation is promptly and safely discarded. Immediate-use compounded sterile preparations shall not be stored for later use
- Cytotoxic drugs shall not be prepared as immediate-use compounded sterile preparations

Environment

A pharmacy that prepares low- and medium-risk preparations shall have a clean room/controlled area for the compounding of sterile preparations that is constructed to minimize the opportunities for particulate and microbial contamination. The clean room/controlled area shall
- Contain an anteroom/ante-zone that provides at least an ISO Class 8 air quality
- Contain a buffer zone or buffer room designed to maintain at least ISO Class 7 conditions

The pharmacy shall prepare sterile pharmaceuticals in a primary engineering control device, such as a laminar air flow hood, biological safety cabinet, compounding aseptic isolator, compounding aseptic containment isolator which is capable of maintaining at least ISO Class 5 conditions during normal activity. The isolator must provide isolation from the room and maintain ISO Class 5 during dynamic operating conditions, including transferring ingredients, components, and devices into and out of the isolator and during preparation of compounded sterile preparations

Cytotoxic Drugs
- All personnel involved in the compounding of cytotoxic products shall wear appropriate protective apparel, such as gowns, face masks, eye protection, hair covers, shoe covers or dedicated shoes, and appropriate gloving
- Cytotoxic drugs shall be prepared in a Class II or III vertical flow biological safety cabinet or compounding aseptic containment isolator located in an ISO Class 7 area that is physically separated from other preparation areas
- Compounding area must have negative air pressure compared to the anteroom, which must have positive air pressure

Cleaning and Disinfecting the Sterile Compounding Areas
- Shall be conducted prior to and after each work shift (at a minimum of every 12 hours while the pharmacy is open) and when there are spills
- Before compounding is performed, all items are removed from the direct and contiguous compounding areas and all surfaces are cleaned of loose material and residue from spills, followed by an application of a residue-free disinfecting agent (e.g., IPA), that is left on for a time sufficient to exert its antimicrobial effect
- Work surfaces near the direct and contiguous compounding areas in the buffer or clean area are cleaned of loose material and residue from spills, followed by an application of a residue-free disinfecting agent that is left on for a time sufficient to exert its antimicrobial effect
- Floors in the buffer or clean area are cleaned by mopping at least once daily when no aseptic operations are in progress

- In the anteroom area, walls, ceilings, and shelving shall be cleaned monthly
- Supplies and equipment removed from shipping cartons must be wiped with a disinfecting agent, such as IPA. No shipping or other external cartons may be taken into the buffer or clean area
- Storage shelving, emptied of all supplies, walls, and ceilings are cleaned and disinfected at least monthly

Personnel Cleansing and Garbing
- Any person with an apparent illness or open lesion that may adversely affect the safety or quality of a drug preparation being compounded shall be excluded from direct contact with components, drug preparation containers, closures, any materials involved in the compounding process, and drug products until the condition is corrected
- Before entering the clean area, compounding personnel must remove the following:
    - personal outer garments (e.g., bandanas, coats, hats, jackets, scarves, sweaters, vests)
    - all cosmetics, because they shed flakes and particles; **and**
    - all hand, wrist, and other body jewelry
- Artificial nails or extenders are prohibited while working in the sterile compounding environment
- Personnel must don personal protective equipment and perform hand hygiene in an order that proceeds from the dirtiest to the cleanest activities as follows:
    - Shoe covers
    - Head and facial hair covers
    - Face mask
    - Wash hands and arms up to elbows – minimum 30 seconds
    - Gown

- Gloves
- 70% IPA to gloves (and routinely during compounding)
- When taking a break – the gown may be stored in the anteroom and reused, but shoe covers, hair and facial hair covers, face mask, and gloves must be replaced, and hand hygiene must be performed

Section Five: Pseudoephederine Laws

Federal

- Sold for personal use through face-to-face stores, mobile retail vendors, or through the mail
- Nonliquid (includes gelcaps) forms **must** be in unit dose packaging
- Report losses to the DEA (examples: theft, in-transit)
- Max of 3.6 grams per day per purchaser
- Max of 7.5 grams per 30-day period per purchaser at a mobile retail vendor
- Customers may not have direct access to the products (e.g., store behind counter or in locked case)
- Seller must maintain a written (bound record book) or electronic list of each sale, including
  - Name of product
  - Quantity sold
  - Name of purchaser
  - Address of purchaser
  - Date and time of sale
  - Signature of purchaser
- Seller must keep the logbook for at least 2 years from the date of sale
- Each seller must do a self-certification with the DEA
- Sales personnel must be trained

Florida

- Max in a single day to an individual = 3.6 grams
- Max of 3 packages in any single, retail, over-the-counter sale
- Max in a 30 day period = 9 grams

- Must be behind a checkout counter where the public is not permitted or other such location that is not otherwise accessible to the general public
- Must have an employee training program
- In order to purchase:
    - Be at least 18 years of age
    - Have government-issued photo identification showing his or her name, date of birth, address, and photo identification number
    - Sign his or her name on a record of the purchase, either on paper or on an electronic signature capture device.
- Allowed to use an electronic recordkeeping system that records:
    - The date and time of the transaction
    - The name, date of birth, address, and photo identification number of the purchaser, as well as the type of identification and the government of issuance.
    - The number of packages purchased, the total grams per package, and the name of the compound, mixture, or preparation containing ephedrine or related compounds.
    - The signature of the purchaser, or a unique number relating the transaction to a paper signature maintained at the retail premises.
- Must keep data for at least 2 years

Section Six: Florida Comprehensive Drug Abuse Prevention and Control Act

Definitions

Administer means the direct application of a controlled substance, whether by injection, inhalation, ingestion, or any other means, to the body of a person or animal.

Controlled substance means any substance named or described in Schedules I-V. Laws controlling the manufacture, distribution, preparation, dispensing, or administration of such substances are drug abuse laws.

Deliver or **delivery** means the actual, constructive, or attempted transfer from one person to another of a controlled substance, whether or not there is an agency relationship.

Dispense means the transfer of possession of one or more doses of a medicinal drug by a pharmacist or other licensed practitioner to the ultimate consumer thereof or to one who represents that it is his or her intention not to consume or use the same but to transfer the same to the ultimate consumer or user for consumption by the ultimate consumer or user.

Distribute means to deliver, other than by administering or dispensing, a controlled substance.

Distributor means a person who distributes.

Department means the Department of Health.

Hospital means an institution for the care and treatment of the sick and injured, licensed pursuant to the provisions of chapter 395 or owned or operated by the state or Federal Government.

Laboratory means a laboratory approved by the Drug Enforcement Administration as proper to be entrusted with the custody of controlled substances for scientific, medical, or instructional purposes or to aid law enforcement officers and prosecuting attorneys in the enforcement of this chapter.

Manufacture means the production, preparation, propagation, compounding, cultivating, growing, conversion, or processing of a controlled substance, either directly or indirectly, by extraction from substances of natural origin, or independently by means of chemical synthesis, or by a combination of extraction and chemical synthesis, and includes any packaging of the substance or labeling or relabeling of its container, except that this term does not include the preparation, compounding, packaging, or labeling of a controlled substance by:

- A practitioner or pharmacist as an incident to his or her administering or delivering of a controlled substance in the course of his or her professional practice.
- A practitioner, or by his or her authorized agent under the practitioner's supervision, for the purpose of, or as an incident to, research, teaching, or chemical analysis, and not for sale.

Manufacturer means and includes every person who prepares, derives, produces, compounds, or repackages any drug as defined by the Florida Drug and Cosmetic Act. However, this definition does not apply to manufacturers of patent or proprietary preparations as defined in the Florida Pharmacy Act. Pharmacies, and pharmacists employed thereby, are specifically excluded from this definition.

Mixture means any physical combination of two or more substances.

Patient means an individual to whom a controlled substance is lawfully dispensed or administered pursuant to the provisions of this chapter.

Pharmacist means a person who is licensed pursuant to chapter 465 to practice the profession of pharmacy in this state.

Possession includes temporary possession for the purpose of verification or testing, irrespective of dominion or control.

Potential for abuse means that a substance has properties of a central nervous system stimulant or depressant or an hallucinogen that create a substantial likelihood of its being:
- Used in amounts that create a hazard to the user's health or the safety of the community;
- Diverted from legal channels and distributed through illegal channels; or
- Taken on the user's own initiative rather than on the basis of professional medical advice.

Practitioner means a physician licensed pursuant to chapter 458, a dentist licensed pursuant to chapter 466, a veterinarian licensed pursuant to chapter 474, an osteopathic physician licensed pursuant to chapter 459, a naturopath licensed pursuant to chapter 462, or a podiatric physician licensed pursuant to chapter 461, provided such practitioner holds a valid federal controlled substance registry number.

Prescription means and includes an order for drugs or medicinal supplies written, signed, or transmitted by word of mouth, telephone, telegram, or other means of communication by a duly licensed practitioner licensed by the laws of the state to prescribe such drugs or medicinal supplies, issued in good faith and in the course of professional practice, intended to be filled, compounded, or dispensed by another person licensed by the laws of the state to do so, and meeting the requirements of s. 893.04. The term also includes an order for drugs or medicinal supplies so transmitted or written by a physician, dentist, veterinarian, or other practitioner licensed to practice in a state other than Florida, but only if the pharmacist called upon to fill such an order determines, in the exercise of his or her professional judgment, that the order was issued pursuant to a valid patient-physician relationship, that it is authentic, and that the drugs or medicinal supplies so ordered are considered necessary for the continuation of treatment of a chronic or recurrent illness. However, if the physician writing the prescription is not known to the pharmacist, the pharmacist shall obtain proof to a reasonable certainty of the validity of said prescription.

Wholesaler means any person who acts as a jobber, wholesale merchant, or broker, or an agent thereof, who sells or distributes for resale any drug as defined by the Florida Drug and Cosmetic Act. However, this definition does not apply to persons who sell only patent or proprietary preparations as defined in the Florida Pharmacy Act. Pharmacies, and pharmacists employed thereby, are specifically excluded from this definition.

Standards and Schedules

SCHEDULE I.—A substance in Schedule I has a high potential for abuse and has no currently accepted medical use in treatment in the United States and in its use under medical supervision does not meet accepted safety standards. Examples: canabis, LSD, heroin, peyote, GHB.

SCHEDULE II.—A substance in Schedule II has a high potential for abuse and has a currently accepted but severely restricted medical use in treatment in the United States, and abuse of the substance may lead to severe psychological or physical dependence. Examples: opium, codeine, hydrocodone, hydromorphone, morphine, oxycodone, cocaine, fentanyl, methadone, meperidine, PCP, sufentanil, amphetamine, methylphenidate, pentobarbital.

SCHEDULE III.—A substance in Schedule III has a potential for abuse less than the substances contained in Schedules I and II and has a currently accepted medical use in treatment in the United States, and abuse of the substance may lead to moderate or low physical dependence or high psychological dependence or, in the case of anabolic steroids, may lead to physical damage. Examples: any derivative of barbituric acid, anabolic steroids including testosterone, ketamine, dronabinol.
- Not more than 1.8 grams of codeine per 100 milliliters or not more than 90 milligrams per dosage unit, with an equal or greater quantity of an isoquinoline alkaloid of opium
- Not more than 1.8 grams of codeine per 100 milliliters or not more than 90 milligrams per dosage unit, with recognized therapeutic amounts of one or more active ingredients which are not controlled substances
- Not more than 300 milligrams of hydrocodone per 100 milliliters or not more than 15 milligrams per dosage unit, with a fourfold or greater quantity of an isoquinoline alkaloid of opium
- Not more than 300 milligrams of hydrocodone per 100 milliliters or not more than 15 milligrams per dosage unit, with recognized therapeutic amounts of one or more active ingredients that are not controlled substances
- Not more than 1.8 grams of dihydrocodeine per 100 milliliters or not more than 90 milligrams per dosage unit, with recognized therapeutic amounts of one or more active ingredients which are not controlled substances
- Not more than 50 milligrams of morphine per 100 milliliters or per 100 grams, with recognized therapeutic amounts of one or more active ingredients which are not controlled substances

SCHEDULE IV.—A substance in Schedule IV has a low potential for abuse relative to the substances in Schedule III and has a currently accepted medical use in treatment in the United States, and abuse of the substance may lead to limited physical or psychological dependence relative to the substances in Schedule III. Examples: Benzodiazepams, Phenobarbital, phentermine, carisoprodol.

SCHEDULE V.—A substance, compound, mixture, or preparation of a substance in Schedule V has a low potential for abuse relative to the substances in Schedule IV and has a currently accepted medical use in treatment in the United States, and abuse of such compound, mixture, or preparation may lead to limited physical or psychological dependence relative to the substances in Schedule IV.
- Not more than 200 milligrams of codeine per 100 milliliters or per 100 grams
- Not more than 100 milligrams of dihydrocodeine per 100 milliliters or per 100 grams
- Not more than 100 milligrams of ethylmorphine per 100 milliliters or per 100 grams
- Not more than 2.5 milligrams of diphenoxylate and not less than 25 micrograms of atropine sulfate per dosage unit
- Not more than 100 milligrams of opium per 100 milliliters or per 100 grams

Scheduling Controlled Substances
The Attorney General may add a substance to a schedule, transfer a substance between schedules, or remove a substance from a schedule.

Controlled Substance Prescriptions
- Cannot have controlled substances from different classes on the same prescription blank
- A controlled substance cannot be on the same prescription blank as a medicinal drug (not a controlled substance)

Out of State Controlled Substance Prescriptions
May fill a prescription for a drug from a physician, dentist, veterinarian, or other practitioner licensed to practice in a state other than Florida, but only if the pharmacist determines, in the exercise of his or her professional judgment, that the order was:
- Issued pursuant to a valid patient-physician relationship, that it is authentic
- Drugs or medicinal supplies so ordered are considered necessary for the continuation of treatment of a chronic or recurrent illness.

However, if the physician writing the prescription is not known to the pharmacist, the pharmacist shall obtain proof to a reasonable certainty of the validity of said prescription.

Controlled Substance Prescriptions
A pharmacist may dispense controlled substances upon a written or oral prescription of a practitioner, under the following conditions:
- Oral prescriptions must be promptly reduced to writing by the pharmacist or recorded electronically if permitted by federal law.
- The written prescription must be dated and signed by the prescribing practitioner on the day when issued.

Controlled Substance Prescription Requirements
- The full name and address of the person for whom, or the owner of the animal for which, the controlled substance is dispensed.
- The full name and address of the prescribing practitioner and the practitioner's federal controlled substance registry number shall be printed thereon.
- If the prescription is for an animal, the species of animal for which the controlled substance is prescribed.
- The name of the controlled substance prescribed and the strength, quantity, and directions for use thereof.

- The number of the prescription, as recorded in the prescription files of the pharmacy in which it is filled.
- The initials of the pharmacist filling the prescription and the date filled.
- The prescription shall be retained on file by the proprietor of the pharmacy in which it is filled for a period of 2 years.

Controlled Substance Prescription Label Requirements
- The name and address of the pharmacy from which such controlled substance was dispensed.
- The date on which the prescription for such controlled substance was filled.
- The number of such prescription, as recorded in the prescription files of the pharmacy in which it is filled.
- The name of the prescribing practitioner.
- The name of the patient for whom, or of the owner and species of the animal for which, the controlled substance is prescribed.
- The directions for the use of the controlled substance prescribed in the prescription.
- A clear, concise warning that it is a crime to transfer the controlled substance to any person other than the patient for whom prescribed.

Schedule II Prescriptions
- Schedule II prescriptions must be written except in an emergency situation where it may be dispensed upon oral prescription but is limited to a 72-hour supply.
- A prescription for a controlled substance listed in Schedule II may not be refilled.

Controlled Substance Prescriptions
- A prescription for a Schedule III, Schedule IV, or Schedule V may not be filled or refilled more than five times within

- a period of 6 months after the date on which the prescription was written
- Pharmacist must make sure prescription is valid before dispensing
- Must obtain suitable identification from the patient prior to dispensing a Schedule II-IV however exempt if dispensed by mail and the patient has insurance
- Can take an oral prescription for a Schedule III or IV, as long as the pharmacist writes it down or records electronically
- For Schedule II-IV must have the quantity written out and numerically noted AND must have the abbreviated month written out on the prescription
- If prescriber not available to verify prescription, then can dispense to patient with valid photographic identification
- If quantity or date not written out in textual format, pharmacist may dispense without verification if they have dispensed to that patient before
- Maximum of 30-day supply of a Schedule III upon an oral prescription issued in this state
- Cannot knowingly fill a forged prescription for a controlled substance
- One time emergency refill up to a 72-hour supply is allowed for any drug other than a Schedule II

Dispensing by a Practitioner
- Practitioner or veterinarian is allowed to prescribe, administer, dispense, mix or prepare a controlled substance
- Must be labeled
    - Date of delivery
    - Directions for use of such controlled substance
    - Name and address of such practitioner
    - Name of the patient and, if such controlled substance is prescribed for an animal, a statement describing the species of the animal

- A clear, concise warning that it is a crime to transfer the controlled substance to any person other than the patient for whom prescribed

Prescription Labeling
- Advanced registered nurse practitioners and physician assistants may prescribe drugs that are not controlled substances as long as they are under the supervision of a licensed practitioner.
- Must include the supervising practitioner's name and professional license number on the prescription and on the dispensed drug container.

Treatment Programs for Impaired Practitioners
- For professions that do not have impaired practitioner programs provided for in their practice acts, the department shall, by rule, designate approved impaired practitioner programs under this section. The department may adopt rules setting forth appropriate criteria for approval of treatment providers. The rules may specify the manner in which the consultant, retained as set forth in subsection (2), works with the department in intervention, requirements for evaluating and treating a professional, requirements for continued care of impaired professionals by approved treatment providers, continued monitoring by the consultant of the care provided by approved treatment providers regarding the professionals under their care, and requirements related to the consultant's expulsion of professionals from the program.
- The department shall retain one or more impaired practitioner consultants. The consultant shall be a licensee under the jurisdiction of the Division of Medical Quality Assurance within the department who must be a practitioner or recovered practitioner licensed under chapter 458, chapter 459, or part I of chapter 464, or an

entity employing a medical director who must be a practitioner or recovered practitioner licensed under chapter 458, chapter 459, or part I of chapter 464. The consultant shall assist the probable cause panel and department in carrying out the responsibilities of this section. This shall include working with department investigators to determine whether a practitioner is, in fact, impaired. The consultant may contract for services to be provided, for appropriate compensation, if requested by the school, for students enrolled in schools for licensure as allopathic physicians or physician assistants under chapter 458, osteopathic physicians or physician assistants under chapter 459, nurses under chapter 464, or pharmacists under chapter 465 who are alleged to be impaired as a result of the misuse or abuse of alcohol or drugs, or both, or due to a mental or physical condition. The department is not responsible under any circumstances for paying the costs of care provided by approved treatment providers, and the department is not responsible for paying the costs of consultants' services provided for students. A medical school accredited by the Liaison Committee on Medical Education of the Commission on Osteopathic College Accreditation, or other school providing for the education of students enrolled in preparation for licensure as allopathic physicians under chapter 458 or osteopathic physicians under chapter 459, which is governed by accreditation standards requiring notice and the provision of due process procedures to students, is not liable in any civil action for referring a student to the consultant retained by the department or for disciplinary actions that adversely affect the status of a student when the disciplinary actions are instituted in reasonable reliance on the recommendations, reports, or conclusions provided by such consultant, if the school, in referring the student or taking disciplinary action, adheres to the due process procedures adopted by the applicable

accreditation entities and if the school committed no intentional fraud in carrying out the provisions of this section.
- Whenever the department receives a written or oral legally sufficient complaint alleging that a licensee under the jurisdiction of the Division of Medical Quality Assurance within the department is impaired as a result of the misuse or abuse of alcohol or drugs, or both, or due to a mental or physical condition which could affect the licensee's ability to practice with skill and safety, and no complaint against the licensee other than impairment exists, the reporting of such information shall not constitute grounds for discipline pursuant to s. 456.072 or the corresponding grounds for discipline within the applicable practice act if the probable cause panel of the appropriate board, or the department when there is no board, finds:
    - The licensee has acknowledged the impairment problem.
    - The licensee has voluntarily enrolled in an appropriate, approved treatment program.
    - The licensee has voluntarily withdrawn from practice or limited the scope of practice as required by the consultant, in each case, until such time as the panel, or the department when there is no board, is satisfied the licensee has successfully completed an approved treatment program.
    - The licensee has executed releases for medical records, authorizing the release of all records of evaluations, diagnoses, and treatment of the licensee, including records of treatment for emotional or mental conditions, to the consultant. The consultant shall make no copies or reports of records that do not regard the issue of the licensee's impairment and his or her participation in a treatment program.

- If, however, the department has not received a legally sufficient complaint and the licensee agrees to withdraw from practice until such time as the consultant determines the licensee has satisfactorily completed an approved treatment program or evaluation, the probable cause panel, or the department when there is no board, shall not become involved in the licensee's case.
- Inquiries related to impairment treatment programs designed to provide information to the licensee and others and which do not indicate that the licensee presents a danger to the public shall not constitute a complaint within the meaning of s. 456.073 and shall be exempt from the provisions of this subsection.
- Whenever the department receives a legally sufficient complaint alleging that a licensee is impaired as described in paragraph (a) and no complaint against the licensee other than impairment exists, the department shall forward all information in its possession regarding the impaired licensee to the consultant. For the purposes of this section, a suspension from hospital staff privileges due to the impairment does not constitute a complaint.
- The probable cause panel, or the department when there is no board, shall work directly with the consultant, and all information concerning a practitioner obtained from the consultant by the panel, or the department when there is no board, shall remain confidential and exempt from the provisions of s. 119.07(1), subject to the provisions of subsections (5) and (6).
- A finding of probable cause shall not be made as long as the panel, or the department when there is no board, is satisfied, based upon information it receives from the consultant and the department, that the licensee is progressing satisfactorily in an approved impaired practitioner program and no other complaint against the licensee exists.
- In any disciplinary action for a violation other than impairment in which a licensee establishes the violation

for which the licensee is being prosecuted was due to or connected with impairment and further establishes the licensee is satisfactorily progressing through or has successfully completed an approved treatment program pursuant to this section, such information may be considered by the board, or the department when there is no board, as a mitigating factor in determining the appropriate penalty. This subsection does not limit mitigating factors the board may consider.

- An approved treatment provider shall, upon request, disclose to the consultant all information in its possession regarding the issue of a licensee's impairment and participation in the treatment program. All information obtained by the consultant and department pursuant to this section is confidential and exempt from the provisions of s. 119.07(1), subject to the provisions of this subsection and subsection (6). Failure to provide such information to the consultant is grounds for withdrawal of approval of such program or provider.
- If in the opinion of the consultant, after consultation with the treatment provider, an impaired licensee has not progressed satisfactorily in a treatment program, all information regarding the issue of a licensee's impairment and participation in a treatment program in the consultant's possession shall be disclosed to the department. Such disclosure shall constitute a complaint pursuant to the general provisions of s. 456.073. Whenever the consultant concludes that impairment affects a licensee's practice and constitutes an immediate, serious danger to the public health, safety, or welfare, that conclusion shall be communicated to the State Surgeon General.
- A consultant, licensee, or approved treatment provider who makes a disclosure pursuant to this section is not subject to civil liability for such disclosure or its consequences. The provisions of s. 766.101 apply to any officer, employee, or agent of the department or the

board and to any officer, employee, or agent of any entity with which the department has contracted pursuant to this section.
- A consultant retained pursuant to subsection (2), a consultant's officers and employees, and those acting at the direction of the consultant for the limited purpose of an emergency intervention on behalf of a licensee or student as described in subsection (2) when the consultant is unable to perform such intervention shall be considered agents of the department for purposes of s. 768.28 while acting within the scope of the consultant's duties under the contract with the department if the contract complies with the requirements of this section. The contract must require that:
    - The consultant indemnify the state for any liabilities incurred up to the limits set out in chapter 768.
    - The consultant establish a quality assurance program to monitor services delivered under the contract.
    - The consultant's quality assurance program, treatment, and monitoring records be evaluated quarterly.
    - The consultant's quality assurance program be subject to review and approval by the department.
    - The consultant operate under policies and procedures approved by the department.
    - The consultant provide to the department for approval a policy and procedure manual that comports with all statutes, rules, and contract provisions approved by the department.
    - The department be entitled to review the records relating to the consultant's performance under the contract for the purpose of management audits, financial audits, or program evaluation.

- - All performance measures and standards be subject to verification and approval by the department.
  - The department be entitled to terminate the contract with the consultant for noncompliance with the contract.
- In accordance with s. 284.385, the Department of Financial Services shall defend any claim, suit, action, or proceeding against the consultant, the consultant's officers or employees, or those acting at the direction of the consultant for the limited purpose of an emergency intervention on behalf of a licensee or student as described in subsection (2) when the consultant is unable to perform such intervention which is brought as a result of any act or omission by any of the consultant's officers and employees and those acting under the direction of the consultant for the limited purpose of an emergency intervention on behalf of a licensee or student as described in subsection (2) when the consultant is unable to perform such intervention when such act or omission arises out of and in the scope of the consultant's duties under its contract with the department.
- If the consultant retained pursuant to subsection (2) is retained by any other state agency, and if the contract between such state agency and the consultant complies with the requirements of this section, the consultant, the consultant's officers and employees, and those acting under the direction of the consultant for the limited purpose of an emergency intervention on behalf of a licensee or student as described in subsection (2) when the consultant is unable to perform such intervention shall be considered agents of the state for the purposes of this section while acting within the scope of and pursuant to guidelines established in the contract between such state agency and the consultant.

Written Prescriptions for Medicinal Drugs
- Written or electronically submitted prescriptions must have/contain:
    - Legibly printed or typed
    - Name of prescribing practitioner
    - Name and strength of the drug prescribed
    - Quantity of the drug prescribed
    - Directions for use of the drug
    - Dated
    - Signed by the prescribing practitioner on the day when issued
- A written prescription for a controlled substance must have:
    - Quantity of the drug prescribed in both textual and numerical formats
    - Dated with the abbreviated month written out on the face of the prescription
    - Written on a standardized counterfeit-proof prescription pad or electronically prescribed

Controlled Substance Prescribing for the Treatment of Chronic Nonmalignant Pain
DEFINITIONS.
- "Addiction medicine specialist" means a board-certified psychiatrist with a subspecialty certification in addiction medicine or who is eligible for such subspecialty certification in addiction medicine, an addiction medicine physician certified or eligible for certification by the American Society of Addiction Medicine, or an osteopathic physician who holds a certificate of added qualification in Addiction Medicine through the American Osteopathic Association.
- "Board-certified pain management physician" means a physician who possesses board certification in pain medicine by the American Board of Pain Medicine, board certification by the American Board of Interventional

Pain Physicians, or board certification or subcertification in pain management or pain medicine by a specialty board recognized by the American Association of Physician Specialists or the American Board of Medical Specialties or an osteopathic physician who holds a certificate in Pain Management by the American Osteopathic Association.
- "Board eligible" means successful completion of an anesthesia, physical medicine and rehabilitation, rheumatology, or neurology residency program approved by the Accreditation Council for Graduate Medical Education or the American Osteopathic Association for a period of 6 years from successful completion of such residency program.
- "Chronic nonmalignant pain" means pain unrelated to cancer which persists beyond the usual course of disease or the injury that is the cause of the pain or more than 90 days after surgery

REGISTRATION
- A licensed physician who prescribes any controlled substance, listed in Schedule II, Schedule III, or Schedule IV for the treatment of chronic nonmalignant pain, must designate himself or herself as a controlled substance prescribing practitioner on the physician's practitioner profile.

STANDARDS OF PRACTICE
- A complete medical history and a physical examination must be conducted before beginning any treatment and must be documented in the medical record. The exact components of the physical examination shall be left to the judgment of the clinician who is expected to perform a physical examination proportionate to the diagnosis that justifies a treatment. The medical record must, at a minimum, document the nature and intensity of the pain, current and past treatments for pain, underlying or coexisting diseases or conditions, the effect of the pain on physical and psychological function, a review of previous

medical records, previous diagnostic studies, and history of alcohol and substance abuse. The medical record shall also document the presence of one or more recognized medical indications for the use of a controlled substance. Each registrant must develop a written plan for assessing each patient's risk of aberrant drug-related behavior, which may include patient drug testing. Registrants must assess each patient's risk for aberrant drug-related behavior and monitor that risk on an ongoing basis in accordance with the plan.

- Each registrant must develop a written individualized treatment plan for each patient. The treatment plan shall state objectives that will be used to determine treatment success, such as pain relief and improved physical and psychosocial function, and shall indicate if any further diagnostic evaluations or other treatments are planned. After treatment begins, the physician shall adjust drug therapy to the individual medical needs of each patient. Other treatment modalities, including a rehabilitation program, shall be considered depending on the etiology of the pain and the extent to which the pain is associated with physical and psychosocial impairment. The interdisciplinary nature of the treatment plan shall be documented.
- The physician shall discuss the risks and benefits of the use of controlled substances, including the risks of abuse and addiction, as well as physical dependence and its consequences, with the patient, persons designated by the patient, or the patient's surrogate or guardian if the patient is incompetent. The physician shall use a written controlled substance agreement between the physician and the patient outlining the patient's responsibilities, including, but not limited to:
    - Number and frequency of controlled substance prescriptions and refills.

- - Patient compliance and reasons for which drug therapy may be discontinued, such as a violation of the agreement.
  - An agreement that controlled substances for the treatment of chronic nonmalignant pain shall be prescribed by a single treating physician unless otherwise authorized by the treating physician and documented in the medical record.
- The patient shall be seen by the physician at regular intervals, not to exceed 3 months, to assess the efficacy of treatment, ensure that controlled substance therapy remains indicated, evaluate the patient's progress toward treatment objectives, consider adverse drug effects, and review the etiology of the pain. Continuation or modification of therapy shall depend on the physician's evaluation of the patient's progress. If treatment goals are not being achieved, despite medication adjustments, the physician shall reevaluate the appropriateness of continued treatment. The physician shall monitor patient compliance in medication usage, related treatment plans, controlled substance agreements, and indications of substance abuse or diversion at a minimum of 3-month intervals.
- The physician shall refer the patient as necessary for additional evaluation and treatment in order to achieve treatment objectives. Special attention shall be given to those patients who are at risk for misusing their medications and those whose living arrangements pose a risk for medication misuse or diversion. The management of pain in patients with a history of substance abuse or with a comorbid psychiatric disorder requires extra care, monitoring, and documentation and requires consultation with or referral to an addiction medicine specialist or psychiatrist.
- A physician registered under this section must maintain accurate, current, and complete records that are accessible and readily available for review and comply

with the requirements of this section, the applicable practice act, and applicable board rules. The medical records must include, but are not limited to:
- The complete medical history and a physical examination, including history of drug abuse or dependence.
- Diagnostic, therapeutic, and laboratory results.
- Evaluations and consultations.
- Treatment objectives.
- Discussion of risks and benefits.
- Treatments.
- Medications, including date, type, dosage, and quantity prescribed.
- Instructions and agreements.
- Periodic reviews.
- Results of any drug testing.
- A photocopy of the patient's government-issued photo identification.
- If a written prescription for a controlled substance is given to the patient, a duplicate of the prescription.
- The physician's full name presented in a legible manner.

- Patients with signs or symptoms of substance abuse shall be immediately referred to a board-certified pain management physician, an addiction medicine specialist, or a mental health addiction facility as it pertains to drug abuse or addiction unless the physician is board-certified or board-eligible in pain management. Throughout the period of time before receiving the consultant's report, a prescribing physician shall clearly and completely document medical justification for continued treatment with controlled substances and those steps taken to ensure medically appropriate use of controlled substances by the patient. Upon receipt of the consultant's written report, the prescribing physician shall incorporate the consultant's recommendations for continuing, modifying, or discontinuing controlled substance therapy. The resulting changes in treatment shall be specifically documented in the patient's medical record. Evidence or behavioral indications of diversion shall be followed by discontinuation of controlled substance therapy, and the patient shall be discharged, and all results of testing and actions taken by the physician shall be documented in the patient's medical record.

This subsection does not apply to a board-eligible or board-certified anesthesiologist, physiatrist, rheumatologist, or neurologist, or to a board-certified physician who has surgical privileges at a hospital or ambulatory surgery center and primarily provides surgical services. This subsection does not apply to a board-eligible or board-certified medical specialist who has also completed a fellowship in pain medicine approved by the Accreditation Council for Graduate Medical Education or the American Osteopathic Association, or who is board eligible or board certified in pain medicine by the American Board of Pain Medicine or a board approved by the American Board of Medical Specialties or the American Osteopathic Association and performs interventional pain procedures of the type routinely billed using surgical codes. This subsection does not apply to a physician who prescribes medically necessary controlled substances for a patient during an inpatient stay in a hospital licensed.

Section Seven: Florida Law Chapter 465 - Pharmacy

Definitions

Administration – means the obtaining and giving of a single dose of medicinal drugs by a legally authorized person to a patient for her or his consumption

Board – the Board of Pharmacy

Consultant pharmacist – a pharmacist licensed by the department and certified as a consultant pharmacist

Data communication device – an electronic device that receives electronic information from one source and transmits or routes it to another, including, but not limited to, any such bridge, router, switch, or gateway

Department – the Department of Health

Dispense – the transfer of possession of one or more doses of a medicinal drug by a pharmacist to the ultimate consumer or her or his agent. As an element of dispensing, the pharmacist shall, prior to the actual physical transfer, interpret and assess the prescription order for potential adverse reactions, interactions, and dosage regimen she or he deems appropriate in the exercise of her or his professional judgment, and the pharmacist shall certify that the medicinal drug called for by the prescription is ready for transfer. The pharmacist shall also provide counseling on proper drug usage, either orally or in writing, if in the exercise of her or his professional judgment counseling is necessary. The actual sales transaction and delivery of such drug shall not be considered dispensing. The administration shall not be considered dispensing

Institutional formulary system – a method whereby the medical staff evaluates, appraises, and selects those medicinal drugs or proprietary preparations which in the medical staff's clinical judgment are most useful in patient care, and which are available for dispensing by a practicing pharmacist in a Class II institutional pharmacy

Medicinal drugs or **drugs** – those substances or preparations commonly known as **prescription** or **legend** drugs which are required by federal or state law to be dispensed only on a prescription, but shall not include patents or proprietary preparations as hereafter defined

Patent or proprietary preparation – a medicine in its unbroken, original package which is sold to the public by, or under the authority of, the manufacturer or primary distributor thereof and which is not misbranded under the provisions of the Florida Drug and Cosmetic Act

Pharmacist – any person licensed pursuant to this chapter to practice the profession of pharmacy

Pharmacy – includes a community pharmacy, an institutional pharmacy, a nuclear pharmacy, a special pharmacy, and an Internet pharmacy

Community pharmacy – includes every location where medicinal drugs are compounded, dispensed, stored, or sold or where prescriptions are filled or dispensed on an outpatient basis

Institutional pharmacy – includes every location in a hospital, clinic, nursing home, dispensary, sanitarium, extended care facility, or other facility, hereinafter referred to as **health care institutions**, where medicinal drugs are compounded, dispensed, stored, or sold

Nuclear pharmacy – includes every location where radioactive drugs and chemicals within the classification of medicinal drugs are compounded, dispensed, stored, or sold. The term nuclear pharmacy does not include hospitals licensed under chapter 395 or the nuclear medicine facilities of such hospitals

Special pharmacy – includes every location where medicinal drugs are compounded, dispensed, stored, or sold if such locations are not otherwise defined in this subsection

Internet pharmacy – includes locations not otherwise licensed or issued a permit under this chapter, within or outside this state, which use the Internet to communicate with or obtain information from consumers in this state and use such communication or information to fill or refill prescriptions or to dispense, distribute, or otherwise engage in the practice of pharmacy in this state. Any act described in this definition constitutes the practice of pharmacy.
The pharmacy department of any permittee shall be considered closed whenever a Florida licensed pharmacist is not present and on duty. The term "**not present and on duty**" shall not be construed to prevent a pharmacist from exiting the prescription department for the purposes of consulting or responding to inquiries or providing assistance to patients or customers, attending to personal hygiene needs, or performing any other function for which the pharmacist is responsible, provided that such activities are conducted in a manner consistent with the pharmacist's responsibility to provide pharmacy services.

Pharmacy intern – means a person who is currently registered in, and attending, a duly accredited college or school of pharmacy, or who is a graduate of such a school or college of pharmacy, and who is duly and properly registered with the department as provided for under its rules.

Practice of the profession of pharmacy – includes compounding, dispensing, and consulting concerning contents, therapeutic values, and uses of any medicinal drug; consulting concerning therapeutic values and interactions of patent or proprietary preparations, whether pursuant to prescriptions or in the absence and entirely independent of such prescriptions or orders; and other pharmaceutical services. For purposes of this subsection, "**other pharmaceutical services**" means the monitoring of the patient's drug therapy and assisting the patient in the management of his or her drug therapy, and includes review of the patient's drug therapy and communication with the patient's prescribing health care provider as licensed under chapter 458, chapter 459, chapter 461, or chapter 466, or similar statutory provision in another jurisdiction, or such provider's agent or such other persons as specifically authorized by the patient, regarding the drug therapy. However, nothing in this subsection may be interpreted to permit an alteration of a prescriber's directions, the diagnosis or treatment of any disease, the initiation of any drug therapy, the practice of medicine, or the practice of osteopathic medicine, unless otherwise permitted by law. "**Practice of the profession of pharmacy**" also includes any other act, service, operation, research, or transaction incidental to, or forming a part of, any of the foregoing acts, requiring, involving, or employing the science or art of any branch of the pharmaceutical profession, study, or training, and shall expressly permit a pharmacist to transmit information from persons authorized to prescribe medicinal drugs to their patients. The practice of the profession of pharmacy also includes the administration of influenza virus immunizations to adults pursuant to s. 465.189.

Prescription – includes any order for drugs or medicinal supplies written or transmitted by any means of communication by a duly licensed practitioner authorized by the laws of the state to prescribe such drugs or medicinal supplies and intended to be dispensed by a pharmacist. The term also includes an orally transmitted order by the lawfully designated agent of such practitioner. The term also includes an order written or transmitted by a practitioner licensed to practice in a jurisdiction other than this state, but only if the pharmacist called upon to dispense such order determines, in the exercise of her or his professional judgment, that the order is valid and necessary for the treatment of a chronic or recurrent illness. The term "**prescription**" also includes a pharmacist's order for a product selected from the formulary created pursuant to s. 465.186. Prescriptions may be retained in written form or the pharmacist may cause them to be recorded in a data processing system, provided that such order can be produced in printed form upon lawful request.

Nuclear pharmacist – means a pharmacist licensed by the department and certified as a nuclear pharmacist pursuant to s. 465.0126.

Centralized prescription filling – means the filling of a prescription by one pharmacy upon request by another pharmacy to fill or refill the prescription. The term includes the performance by one pharmacy for another pharmacy of other pharmacy duties such as drug utilization review, therapeutic drug utilization review, claims adjudication, and the obtaining of refill authorizations.

Automated pharmacy system – means a mechanical system that delivers prescription drugs received from a Florida licensed pharmacy and maintains related transaction information.
Sterile Compounding Definitions

Sterile Compounding Definitions

Anteroom means an area where personnel perform hand hygiene and garbing procedures, staging of components, order entry, CSP labeling, and other high-particulate generating activities. It is also a transition area that provides assurance that pressure relationships are constantly maintained so that air flows from clean to dirty areas. The Anteroom area is to be maintained within ISO Class 8 level of particulate contamination.

Antineoplastic means a pharmaceutical agent that has the intent of causing cell death targeted to cancer cells, metastatic cells, or other cells involved in a severe inflammatory or autoimmune response.

Beyond-use-date means the date after which a compounded preparation should not be used and is determined from the date the preparation was compounded.

Biological safety cabinet means a containment unit suitable for the preparation of low, moderate, and high risk agents where there is a need for protection of the product, personnel, and environment.

Bulk Compounding means the compounding of CSPs in increments of twenty-five (25) or more doses from a single source.

Buffer area (Clean room) is an area where the activities of CSP take place; it shall not contain sinks or drains. In High-Risk compounding this must be a separate room. The Buffer area is to be maintained within ISO Class 7 level of particulate contamination.

Class 100 environment means an atmospheric environment which contains no more than one hundred particles of 0.5 microns in diameter or larger per cubic foot of air. A class 100 environment is equivalent to ISO Class 5 level of particulate contamination.

Compounding Aseptic Isolator (CAI) – is a form of barrier isolator specifically designed for compounding pharmaceutical ingredients or preparations. It is designed to maintain an aseptic compounding environment within the isolator throughout the compounding and material transfer process. Air exchange into the isolator from the surrounding environment should not occur unless it is first passed through a microbially retentive filter (HEPA minimum 0.2 microns).

High-Risk Level CSPs – are products compounded under any of the following conditions are either non-sterile or at high risk to become non-sterile with infectious microorganisms.
- Non-sterile ingredients, including manufactured products for routes of administration other than sterile parenteral administration are incorporated or a non-sterile device is employed before terminal sterilization.
- Sterile contents of commercially manufactured products, CSP that lack effective antimicrobial preservatives, sterile surfaces of devices and containers for the preparation, transfer, sterilization, and packaging of CSPs are exposed to air quality worse than ISO Class 5 for more than one (1) hour.
- Before sterilization, non-sterile procedures such as weighing and mixing are conducted in air quality worse than ISO Class 7, compounding personnel are improperly garbed and gloved, or water-containing preparations are stored for more than 6 hours.
- For properly stored sterilized high-risk preparation, in the absence of passing a sterility test, the storage periods cannot exceed the following time periods: before administration, the CSPs are properly stored and exposed for not more than 24 hours at controlled room temperature, and for not more than 3 days at a cold temperature (2-8 degrees Celsius) and for not more than 45 days in solid frozen state at -20 degrees celsius or colder.
- Examples of high-risk compounding include: (1) dissolving non-sterile bulk drug and nutrient powders to make solutions, which will be terminally sterilized; (2) exposing the sterile ingredients and components used to prepare and package CSPs to room air quality worse than ISO Class 5 for more than one (1) hour; (3) measuring and mixing sterile ingredients in non-sterile devices

before sterilization is performed; (4) assuming, without appropriate evidence or direct determination, that packages of bulk ingredients contain at least 95% by weight of their active chemical moiety and have not been contaminated or adulterated between uses.
- All high risk category products must be rendered sterile by heat sterilization, gas sterilization, or filtration sterilization in order to become a CSP.
- Quality assurance practices for high-risk level CSPs include all those for low-risk level CSPs. In addition, each person authorized to compound high-risk level CSPs demonstrates competency by completing a media-filled test that represents high-level compounding semiannually.

Immediate Use CSPs
- Requires only simple aseptic measuring and transfer manipulations are performed with not more than three (3) sterile non-hazardous drug or diagnostic radiopharmaceutical drug preparations, including an infusion or dilution solution.
- The preparation procedure occurs continuously without delays or interruptions and does not exceed 1 hour.
- At no point during preparation and prior to administration are critical surfaces and ingredients of the CSP directly exposed to contact contamination such as human touch, cosmetic flakes or particulates, blood, human body substances (excretions and secretions, e.g., nasal or oral) and non-sterile inanimate sources.
- Administration begins not later than one (1) hour following the start of preparing the CSP.
- When the CSP is not administered by the person who prepared it, or its administration is not witnessed by the person who prepared it, the CSP container shall bear a label listing patient identification information (name, identification numbers), and the names and amounts of all active ingredients, and the name or identifiable initials

of the person who prepared the CSP, and one (1) hour beyond-use time and date.
- If administration has not begun within one (1) hour following the start of preparing the CSP, the CSP is promptly and safely discarded. Immediate use CSPs shall not be stored for later use.

ISO Class 5 guidelines are met when particulate contamination is measured at "not more than 3,520 particles 0.5 micron size or larger per cubic meter of air for any lamiar airflow workbench (LAWF), BSC, or CAI. (Also referred to as a "Class 100 environment.")

ISO Class 7 guidelines are met when particulate contamination is measured at "not more than 352,000 particles 0.5 micron size or larger per cubic meter of air for any buffer area (room)."

ISO Class 8 guidelines are met when particulate contamination is measured at "not more than 3,520,000 particles 0.5 micron size or larger per cubic meter of air for any anteroom (area)."

Low-Risk Level CSPs compounded under all of the following are at a low risk of contamination:
- The CSPs are compounded with aseptic manipulations entirely within ISO Class 5 (class 100) or better air quality using only sterile ingredients, products, components, and devices.
- The compounding involves only transfer, measuring, and mixing manipulations using no more than three commercially manufactured sterile products and entries into one container (e.g., bag, vial) of sterile product to make the CSP.
- Manipulations are limited to aseptically opening ampoules, penetrating sterile stoppers on vials with sterile needles and syringes, and transferring sterile liquids in sterile syringes to sterile administration devices, package containers for storage and dispensing.

- The contents of ampoules shall be passed through a sterile filter to remove any particles.
- For low-risk preparation, in the absence of passing a sterility test or a documented validated process, the storage periods cannot exceed the following time periods; before administration, the CSPs are properly stored and exposed for not more than 48 hours at controlled room temperature, and for not more than 14 days at a cold temperature (2-8 degrees celsius) and for 45 days in solid frozen state at -20 degrees celsius or colder.
- Quality Assurance practices include, but are not limited to, the following: (1) routine disinfection and air quality testing of the direct compounding environment to minimize microbial surface contamination and maintain ISO Class 5 air quality; (2) Visual confirmation that compounding personnel are properly donning and wearing appropriate items and types of protective garments; (3) Review of all orders and packages of ingredients to ensure that the correct identity and amounts of ingredients were compounded; (4) Visual inspection of CSPs to ensure the absence of particulate matter in solutions, the absence of leakage from vials and bags, and accuracy and thoroughness of labeling.
- All compounding personnel are required to demonstrate competency by completing a media-filled test that represents low-level compounding annually. A media-filled test is a commercially available sterile fluid culture media that shall be able to promote exponential colonization of bacteria that are both likely to be transmitted to CSP from the compounding personnel and environment. Media filled vials are incubated at 25-35 degrees celsius for 14 days. Failure is indicated by visible turbidity in the medium on or before 14 days.

Medium-Risk Level CSPs – When CSPs are compounded aseptically under Low-Risk Conditions, and one or more of the

following conditions exist, such CSPs are at a medium risk of contamination:
- CSPs containing more than three (3) commercial sterile drug products and those requiring complex manipulations and/or preparation methods.
- Multiple individual or small doses of sterile products are combined or pooled to prepare a CSP that will be administered either to multiple patients or to one patient on multiple occasions.
- The compounding process requires unusually long duration, such as that required to complete dissolution or homogeneous mixing.
- For Medium-risk preparation, in the absence of passing a sterility test or a documented validated process, the storage periods cannot exceed the following time periods; before administration, the CSPs are properly stored and exposed for not more than 30 hours at controlled room temperature, and for not more than 9 days at a cold temperature and for 45 days in solid frozen state at -20 degrees celsius or colder.
- These include compounding of total parenteral nutrition (TPN) using either manual or automated devices during which there are multiple injections, detachments, and attachments of nutrient source products to the device or machine to deliver all nutritional components to a final sterile container.
- Filling of reservoirs of injection and infusion devices with more than three (3) sterile drug products and evacuation of air from those reservoirs before the filled devices are dispensed.
- Transfer of volumes from multiple ampules or vials into one or more final sterile containers.
- Quality assurance practices for medium-risk level CSPs include all those for low-risk level CSPs.
- Demonstrates competency by completing a media-filled test that represents medium-level compounding annually.

Parenteral means a sterile preparation of drugs for injection through one or more layers of the skin.

Risk level of the sterile preparation means the level assigned to a sterile product by a pharmacist that represents the probability that the sterile product will be contaminated with microbial organisms, spores, endotoxins, foreign chemicals or other physical matter.

Sterile preparation means any dosage form devoid of viable microorganisms, including but not limited to, parenterals, injectables, ophthalmics, and aqueous inhalant solutions for respiratory treatments.

Board of Pharmacy
- 9 members appointed by the Governor and confirmed by the Senate
- 7 members must be licensed pharmacists
    - Residents of this state
    - Practiced pharmacy in this state for at least 4 years
- One pharmacist must be employed in a community pharmacy and one must be employed in an institutional pharmacy
- Remaining 2 members must be
    - Residents of this state
    - No way connected with the practice of pharmacy, drug manufacturer or wholesaler
- At least one member must be 60 years of age or older
- 4 year terms

Licensure by Examination
- Requirements
    - Must pass the required exams
    - Must be at least 18 years old

- o Receive a degree from an accredited college of pharmacy or passed the FPGEE and completed at least 500 hours in a supervised work activity program within this state under the supervision of a pharmacist licensed by the department, which program is approved by the board
- o Complete an internship program approved by the board – not to exceed 2,080 hours
- May take the exams if waiting for age or intern hours

Licensure by Endorsement
- Requirements
  - o Be at least 18 years old
  - o Received a degree from an accredited college of pharmacy
  - o Complete 2080 internship hours within the past two years prior to application OR submit evidence of active licensed practice of pharmacy in another state for at least two (2) of the immediately preceding five (5) years. Candidates applying by this method must submit 30 hours of board-approved continuing education for the two (2) calendar years preceding the application. (For example, if you are applying for licensure in 2010, you must submit 30 hours of board-approved continuing education earned in 2008 and 2009)
  - o Pass the NAPLEX
  - o Submit application with required fees
  - o Pass the MPJE
- If you do not meet these requirements, you must apply by for licensure by examination. You will be required to take both the NAPLEX® and the Multistate Pharmacy Jurisprudence Examination® (MPJE®) (law exam) when applying by examination unless your NAPLEX® score was transferred to Florida within three (3) years of your exam date

- An applicant licensed in another state for a period in excess of 2 years from the date of application for licensure in this state shall submit a total of at least 30 hours of board-approved continuing education for the 2 calendar years immediately preceding application
- The department may not issue a license by endorsement to any applicant whose license to practice pharmacy has been suspended or revoked in another state or who is currently the subject of any disciplinary proceeding in another state

Renewal of License
- Biennial renewal
- Any person licensed for 50 years or more is exempt from the payment of the renewal or delinquent fee, and shall be issued a lifetime license

Continuing Professional Pharmaceutical Education
- 30 hours required during the 2 years prior to renewal of license
- CE courses must be approved by the board

Reactivation of License
- 15 classroom hours for each year the license was inactive in addition to completion of the number of hours required for renewal on the date the license became inactive

Consultant Pharmacist License
- Responsibilities
    - Maintaining all drug records required by law
    - Establishing drug handling procedures for the safe handling and storage of drugs
    - Ordering and evaluating any laboratory or clinical testing but may only be ordered on patients residing in a nursing home facility and then only

- when authorized by the medical director of the nursing home facility
- Must have completed additional training and qualifications in the practice of institutional pharmacy
- Biennial license renewal

Ordering and Evaluating Laboratory or Clinical Testing
- Performed by a consultant pharmacist or a doctor of pharmacy licensed in FL
- Can order and evaluate any laboratory or clinical testing for persons under the care of a licensed home health agency when, in the judgment of the consultant pharmacist or doctor of pharmacy, such activity is necessary for the proper performance of his or her responsibilities and only when authorized by a practitioner
- Must complete 3 hours of continuing education relating to laboratory and clinical testing as established by the board

Nuclear Pharmacists
- Biennial license renewal
- Responsibilities
    - compounding and the dispensing of nuclear pharmaceuticals
    - maintaining all drug records required by law
    - establishing drug handling procedures for the safe handling and storage of radiopharmaceuticals and medicinal drugs
    - providing the security of the prescription department
    - complying with such other rules as relate to the practice of the profession of pharmacy
- Must have completed such additional training and must demonstrate such additional qualifications in the practice

of nuclear pharmacy as is required by the board by rule in addition to licensure as a registered pharmacist

Pharmacy Interns
- Must be registered with the board
- Enrolled in an intern program at an accredited school or college of pharmacy or who are graduates of accredited schools or colleges of pharmacy and are not yet licensed in the state
- Board may revoke the registration of any intern for good cause, including grounds enumerated in the chapter for revocation of pharmacists' licenses

Pharmacy Technicians
- Must be registered with the board - biennially
- Tasks must be under the direct supervision of a licensed pharmacist
- May initiate or receive communications with a practitioner or his or her agent, on behalf of a patient, regarding refill authorization requests
- A licensed pharmacist may not supervise more than one registered pharmacy technician unless otherwise permitted by the guidelines adopted by the board (maximum of 3 techs)
- Requirements
  - At least 17 years of age
  - Completed a pharmacy technician training program approved by the Board of Pharmacy
- Any registered pharmacy technician registered pursuant to this section before January 1, 2011, who has worked as a pharmacy technician for a minimum of 1,500 hours under the supervision of a licensed pharmacist or received certification as a pharmacy technician by certification program accredited by the National Commission for Certifying Agencies is exempt from the requirement to complete an initial training program for purposes of registration

- A person whose license to practice pharmacy has been denied, suspended, or restricted for disciplinary purposes is not eligible to register as a pharmacy technician
- Notwithstanding the requirements of this section or any other provision of law, a pharmacy technician student who is enrolled in a pharmacy technician training program that is approved by the board may be placed in a pharmacy for the purpose of obtaining practical training. A pharmacy technician student shall wear identification that indicates his or her student status when performing the functions of a pharmacy technician, and registration under this section is not required
- A person who is licensed by the state as a pharmacy intern may be employed as a registered pharmacy technician without paying a registration fee or filing an application with the board to register as a pharmacy technician.
- As a condition of registration renewal, a registered pharmacy technician shall complete 20 hours biennially of continuing education courses approved by the board or the Accreditation Council for Pharmacy Education, of which 4 hours must be via live presentation and 2 hours must be related to the prevention of medication errors and pharmacy law.
- If the board finds that an applicant for registration as a pharmacy technician or that a registered pharmacy technician has committed an act that constitutes grounds for or has committed an act that constitutes grounds for denial of a license or disciplinary action as set forth in this chapter, including an act that constitutes a substantial violation of s. 456.072(1) or a violation of this chapter which occurred before the applicant or registrant was registered as a pharmacy technician, the board may enter an order imposing any of the penalties specified in s. 456.072(2) against the applicant or registrant.

Violations and Penalties
- It is unlawful for any person to own, operate, maintain, open, establish, conduct, or have charge of, either alone or with another person or persons, a pharmacy:
    - Which is not registered under the provisions of this chapter
    - In which a person not licensed as a pharmacist in this state or not registered as an intern in this state or in which an intern who is not acting under the direct and immediate personal supervision of a licensed pharmacist fills, compounds, or dispenses any prescription or dispenses medicinal drugs.
- It is unlawful for any person:
    - To make a false or fraudulent statement, either for herself or himself or for another person, in any application, affidavit, or statement presented to the board or in any proceeding before the board.
    - To fill, compound, or dispense prescriptions or to dispense medicinal drugs if such person does not hold an active license as a pharmacist in this state, is not registered as an intern in this state, or is an intern not acting under the direct and immediate personal supervision of a licensed pharmacist.
    - To sell or dispense drugs as defined in s. 465.003(8) without first being furnished with a prescription.
    - To sell samples or complimentary packages of drug products.
- It is unlawful for any pharmacist to knowingly fail to report to the sheriff or other chief law enforcement agency of the county where the pharmacy is located within 24 hours after learning of any instance in which a person obtained or attempted to obtain a controlled substance, as defined in s. 893.02, or at the close of business on the next business day, whichever is later, that the pharmacist knew or believed was obtained or

attempted to be obtained through fraudulent methods or representations from the pharmacy at which the pharmacist practiced pharmacy. Any pharmacist who knowingly fails to make such a report within 24 hours after learning of the fraud or attempted fraud or at the close of business on the next business day, whichever is later, commits a misdemeanor of the first degree, punishable as provided in s. 775.082 or s. 775.083. A sufficient report of the fraudulent obtaining of controlled substances under this subsection must contain, at a minimum, a copy of the prescription used or presented and a narrative, including all information available to the pharmacist concerning the transaction, such as the name and telephone number of the prescribing physician; the name, description, and any personal identification information pertaining to the person who presented the prescription; and all other material information, such as photographic or video surveillance of the transaction

- It is unlawful for any person other than a pharmacist licensed under this chapter to use the title "pharmacist" or "druggist" or otherwise lead the public to believe that she or he is engaged in the practice of pharmacy.
- It is unlawful for any person other than an owner of a pharmacy registered under this chapter to display any sign or to take any other action that would lead the public to believe that such person is engaged in the business of compounding, dispensing, or retailing any medicinal drugs. This paragraph shall not preclude a person not licensed as a pharmacist from owning a pharmacy
- It is unlawful for a person, firm, or corporation that is not licensed or registered under this chapter to:
    - Use in a trade name, sign, letter, or advertisement any term, including "drug," "pharmacy," "prescription drugs," "Rx," or "apothecary," which implies that the person, firm, or corporation is licensed or registered to practice pharmacy in this state.

- - Hold himself or herself out to others as a person, firm, or corporation licensed or registered to practice pharmacy in this state.
- It is unlawful for a person who is not registered as a pharmacy technician under this chapter or who is not otherwise exempt from the requirement to register as a pharmacy technician, to perform the functions of a registered pharmacy technician, or hold himself or herself out to others as a person who is registered to perform the functions of a registered pharmacy technician in this state.

Registration of Nonresident Pharmacies

- Any pharmacy which is located outside this state and which ships, mails, or delivers, in any manner, a dispensed medicinal drug into this state shall be considered a nonresident pharmacy, shall be registered with the board, shall provide pharmacy services at a high level of protection and competence, and shall disclose to the board the following specific information:
  - That it maintains at all times a valid, unexpired license, permit, or registration to operate the pharmacy in compliance with the laws of the state in which the dispensing facility is located and from which the medicinal drugs shall be dispensed
  - The location, names, and titles of all principal corporate officers and the pharmacist who serves as the prescription department manager for dispensing medicinal drugs to residents of this state. This disclosure shall be made within 30 days after any change of location, corporate officer, or pharmacist serving as the prescription department manager for dispensing medicinal drugs to residents of this state
  - That it complies with all lawful directions and requests for information from the regulatory or licensing agency of all states in which it is licensed

as well as with all requests for information made by the board pursuant to this section. It shall respond directly to all communications from the board concerning emergency circumstances arising from errors in the dispensing of medicinal drugs to the residents of this state
- That it maintains its records of medicinal drugs dispensed to patients in this state so that the records are readily retrievable from the other business records of the pharmacy and from the records of other medicinal drugs dispensed; and
- That during its regular hours of operation but not less than 6 days per week, for a minimum of 40 hours per week, a toll-free telephone service shall be provided to facilitate communication between patients in this state and a pharmacist at the pharmacy who has access to the patient's records. This toll-free number must be disclosed on the label affixed to each container of dispensed medicinal drugs.
- The board may grant an exemption from the registration requirements of this section to any nonresident pharmacy which confines its dispensing activity to isolated transactions. The board may define by rule the term isolated transactions
- The board may deny, revoke, or suspend registration of, or fine or reprimand, a nonresident pharmacy for failure to comply with s. 465.025 or with any requirement of this section in accordance with the provisions of this chapter.
- In addition the board may deny, revoke, or suspend registration of, or fine or reprimand, a nonresident pharmacy in accordance with the provisions of this chapter for conduct which causes serious bodily injury or serious psychological injury to a resident of this state if the board has referred the matter to the regulatory or licensing agency in the state in which the pharmacy is

located and the regulatory or licensing agency fails to investigate within 180 days of the referral.
- It is unlawful for any nonresident pharmacy which is not registered pursuant to this section to advertise its services in this state, or for any person who is a resident of this state to advertise the pharmacy services of a nonresident pharmacy which has not registered with the board, with the knowledge that the advertisement will or is likely to induce members of the public in this state to use the pharmacy to fill prescriptions.
- This section does not apply to Internet pharmacies required to be permitted under s. 465.0197.
- The registered pharmacy and the pharmacist designated by the registered pharmacy as the prescription department manager or the equivalent must be licensed in the state of location in order to dispense into this state.

Disciplinary Actions

The following acts constitute grounds for denial of a license or disciplinary action, as specified in s. 456.072(2):
- Obtaining a license by misrepresentation or fraud or through an error of the department or the board
- Procuring or attempting to procure a license for any other person by making or causing to be made any false representation
- Permitting any person not licensed as a pharmacist in this state or not registered as an intern in this state, or permitting a registered intern who is not acting under the direct and immediate personal supervision of a licensed pharmacist, to fill, compound, or dispense any prescriptions in a pharmacy owned and operated by such pharmacist or in a pharmacy where such pharmacist is employed or on duty.
- Being unfit or incompetent to practice pharmacy by reason of:
  - Habitual intoxication

- - The misuse or abuse of any medicinal drug appearing in any schedule set forth in chapter 893
  - Any abnormal physical or mental condition which threatens the safety of persons to whom she or he might sell or dispense prescriptions, drugs, or medical supplies or for whom she or he might manufacture, prepare, or package, or supervise the manufacturing, preparation, or packaging of, prescriptions, drugs, or medical supplies.
- Violating chapter 499; 21 U.S.C. ss. 301-392, known as the Federal Food, Drug, and Cosmetic Act; 21 U.S.C. ss. 821 et seq., known as the Comprehensive Drug Abuse Prevention and Control Act; or chapter 893.
- Having been convicted or found guilty, regardless of adjudication, in a court of this state or other jurisdiction, of a crime which directly relates to the ability to practice pharmacy or to the practice of pharmacy. A plea of nolo contendere constitutes a conviction for purposes of this provision.
- Using in the compounding of a prescription, or furnishing upon prescription, an ingredient or article different in any manner from the ingredient or article prescribed, except as authorized in s. 465.019(6) or s. 465.025.
- Having been disciplined by a regulatory agency in another state for any offense that would constitute a violation of this chapter.
- Compounding, dispensing, or distributing a legend drug, including any controlled substance, other than in the course of the professional practice of pharmacy. For purposes of this paragraph, it shall be legally presumed that the compounding, dispensing, or distributing of legend drugs in excessive or inappropriate quantities is not in the best interests of the patient and is not in the course of the professional practice of pharmacy.
- Making or filing a report or record which the licensee knows to be false, intentionally or negligently failing to file a report or record required by federal or state law,

willfully impeding or obstructing such filing, or inducing another person to do so. Such reports or records include only those which the licensee is required to make or file in her or his capacity as a licensed pharmacist.
- Failing to make prescription fee or price information readily available by failing to provide such information upon request and upon the presentation of a prescription for pricing or dispensing. Nothing in this section shall be construed to prohibit the quotation of price information on a prescription drug to a potential consumer by telephone.
- Placing in the stock of any pharmacy any part of any prescription compounded or dispensed which is returned by a patient; however, in a hospital, nursing home, correctional facility, or extended care facility in which unit-dose medication is dispensed to inpatients, each dose being individually sealed and the individual unit dose or unit-dose system labeled with the name of the drug, dosage strength, manufacturer's control number, and expiration date, if any, the unused unit dose of medication may be returned to the pharmacy for re-dispensing. Each pharmacist shall maintain appropriate records for any unused or returned medicinal drugs.
- Being unable to practice pharmacy with reasonable skill and safety by reason of illness, use of drugs, narcotics, chemicals, or any other type of material or as a result of any mental or physical condition. A pharmacist affected under this paragraph shall at reasonable intervals be afforded an opportunity to demonstrate that she or he can resume the competent practice of pharmacy with reasonable skill and safety to her or his customers.
- Violating a rule of the board or department or violating an order of the board or department previously entered in a disciplinary hearing.
- Failing to report to the department any licensee under chapter 458 or under chapter 459 who the pharmacist knows has violated the grounds for disciplinary action

set out in the law under which that person is licensed and who provides health care services in a facility licensed under chapter 395, or a health maintenance organization certificated under part I of chapter 641, in which the pharmacist also provides services.
- Failing to notify the Board of Pharmacy in writing within 20 days of the commencement or cessation of the practice of the profession of pharmacy in Florida when such commencement or cessation of the practice of the profession of pharmacy in Florida was a result of a pending or completed disciplinary action or investigation in another jurisdiction.
- Using or releasing a patient's records except as authorized by this chapter and chapter 456.
- Violating any provision of this chapter or chapter 456, or any rules adopted pursuant thereto.
- Dispensing any medicinal drug based upon a communication that purports to be a prescription as defined by s. 465.003(14) or s. 893.02 when the pharmacist knows or has reason to believe that the purported prescription is not based upon a valid practitioner-patient relationship.
- Committing an error or omission during the performance of a specific function of prescription drug processing, which includes, for purposes of this paragraph:
  - Receiving, interpreting, or clarifying a prescription
  - Entering prescription data into the pharmacy's record
  - Verifying or validating a prescription
  - Performing pharmaceutical calculations
  - Performing prospective drug review as defined by the board
  - Obtaining refill and substitution authorizations
  - Interpreting or acting on clinical data
  - Performing therapeutic interventions

- - Providing drug information concerning a patient's prescription
  - Providing patient counseling.
- The board may enter an order denying licensure or imposing any of the penalties in s. 456.072(2) against any applicant for licensure or licensee who is found guilty of violating any provision of subsection (1) of this section or who is found guilty of violating any provision of s. 456.072(1).
- The board shall not reinstate the license of a pharmacist, or cause a license to be issued to a person it has deemed unqualified, until such time as it is satisfied that she or he has complied with all the terms and conditions set forth in the final order and that such person is capable of safely engaging in the practice of pharmacy.

Authority to Inspect

- Duly authorized agents and employees of the department shall have the power to inspect in a lawful manner at all reasonable hours any pharmacy, hospital, clinic, wholesale establishment, manufacturer, physician's office, or any other place in the state in which drugs and medical supplies are manufactured, packed, packaged, made, stored, sold, offered for sale, exposed for sale, or kept for sale for the purpose of:
  - Determining if any of the provisions of this chapter or any rule promulgated under its authority is being violated
  - Securing samples or specimens of any drug or medical supply after paying or offering to pay for such sample or specimen; or
  - Securing such other evidence as may be needed for prosecution under this chapter
- Only a patient or their legal representative may have access to their records. Any civil or criminal proceeding needs a subpoena.

Community Pharmacies; Permits

- Any person desiring a permit to operate a community pharmacy shall apply to the department
- If the board office certifies that the application complies with the laws of the state and the rules of the board governing pharmacies, the department shall issue the permit. No permit shall be issued unless a licensed pharmacist is designated as the prescription department manager
- The board may suspend or revoke the permit of, or may refuse to issue a permit to:
    - Any person who has been disciplined or who has abandoned a permit or allowed a permit to become void after written notice that disciplinary proceedings had been or would be brought against the permit
    - Any person who is an officer, director, or person interested directly or indirectly in a person or business entity that has had a permit disciplined or abandoned or become void after written notice that disciplinary proceedings had been or would be brought against the permit; or
    - Any person who is or has been an officer of a business entity, or who was interested directly or indirectly in a business entity, the permit of which has been disciplined or abandoned or become null and void after written notice that disciplinary proceedings had been or would be brought against the permit.
- In addition to any other remedies provided by law, the board may deny the application or suspend or revoke the license, registration, or certificate of any entity regulated or licensed by it if the applicant, licensee, registrant, or licenseholder, or, in the case of a corporation, partnership, or other business entity, if any officer, director, agent, or managing employee of that business entity or any affiliated person, partner, or shareholder

having an ownership interest equal to 5 percent or greater in that business entity, has failed to pay all outstanding fines, liens, or overpayments assessed by final order of the department, unless a repayment plan is approved by the department, or has failed to comply with any repayment plan.
- Passing an onsite inspection is a prerequisite to the issuance of an initial permit or a permit for a change of location. The department must make the inspection within 90 days before issuance of the permit.
- Community pharmacies that dispense controlled substances must maintain a record of all controlled substance dispensing consistent with the requirements of s. 893.07 and must make the record available to the department and law enforcement agencies upon request.

Institutional Pharmacies; Permits
- Any institution desiring to operate an institutional pharmacy shall apply to the department. If the board certifies that the application complies with the laws of the state and the rules of the board governing pharmacies, the department shall issue the permit.
- The following classes of institutional pharmacies are established:
    - "Class I institutional pharmacies" are those institutional pharmacies in which all medicinal drugs are administered from individual prescription containers to the individual patient and in which medicinal drugs are not dispensed on the premises, except that nursing homes licensed under part II of chapter 400 may purchase medical oxygen for administration to residents. No medicinal drugs may be dispensed in a Class I institutional pharmacy.
    - "Class II institutional pharmacies" are those institutional pharmacies which employ the services of a registered pharmacist or pharmacists

who, in practicing institutional pharmacy, shall provide dispensing and consulting services on the premises to patients of that institution, for use on the premises of that institution. However, an institutional pharmacy located in an area or county included in an emergency order or proclamation of a state of emergency declared by the Governor may provide dispensing and consulting services to individuals who are not patients of the institution. However, a single dose of a medicinal drug may be obtained and administered to a patient on a valid physician's drug order under the supervision of a physician or charge nurse, consistent with good institutional practice procedures. The obtaining and administering of such single dose of a medicinal drug shall be pursuant to drug-handling procedures established by a consultant pharmacist. Medicinal drugs may be dispensed in a Class II institutional pharmacy, but only in accordance with the provisions of this section.
  - "Modified Class II institutional pharmacies" are those institutional pharmacies in short-term, primary care treatment centers that meet all the requirements for a Class II permit, except space and equipment requirements.
- Medicinal drugs shall be stocked, stored, compounded, dispensed, or administered in any health care institution only when that institution has secured an institutional pharmacy permit from the department.
- Medicinal drugs shall be dispensed in an institutional pharmacy to outpatients only when that institution has secured a community pharmacy permit from the department. However, an individual licensed to prescribe medicinal drugs in this state may dispense up to a 24-hour supply of a medicinal drug to any patient of an emergency department of a hospital that operates a Class

II institutional pharmacy, provided that the physician treating the patient in such hospital's emergency department determines that the medicinal drug is warranted and that community pharmacy services are not readily accessible, geographically or otherwise, to the patient. Such dispensing from the emergency department must be in accordance with the procedures of the hospital. For any such patient for whom a medicinal drug is warranted for a period to exceed 24 hours, an individual licensed to prescribe such drug must dispense a 24-hour supply of such drug to the patient and must provide the patient with a prescription for such drug for use after the initial 24-hour period. The board may adopt rules necessary to carry out the provisions of this subsection.

- All institutional pharmacies shall be under the professional supervision of a consultant pharmacist, and the compounding and dispensing of medicinal drugs shall be done only by a licensed pharmacist. Every institutional pharmacy that employs or otherwise uses registered pharmacy technicians shall have a written policy and procedures manual specifying those duties, tasks, and functions that a registered pharmacy technician is allowed to perform.
- In a Class II institutional pharmacy, an institutional formulary system may be adopted with approval of the medical staff for the purpose of identifying those medicinal drugs and proprietary preparations that may be dispensed by the pharmacists employed in such institution. A facility with a Class II institutional permit which is operating under the formulary system shall establish policies and procedures for the development of the system in accordance with the joint standards of the American Hospital Association and American Society of Hospital Pharmacists for the utilization of a hospital formulary system, which formulary shall be approved by the medical staff.

Nuclear Pharmacy Permits

Any person desiring a permit to operate a nuclear pharmacy shall apply to the department. If the board certifies that the application complies with applicable law, the department shall issue the permit. No permit shall be issued unless a duly licensed and qualified nuclear pharmacist is designated as being responsible for activities described in s. 465.0126. The permittee shall notify the department within 10 days of any change of the licensed pharmacist responsible for the compounding and dispensing of nuclear pharmaceuticals.

Special Pharmacy Permits

Any person desiring a permit to operate a special pharmacy shall apply to the department for a special pharmacy permit. If the board certifies that the application complies with the applicable laws and rules of the board governing the practice of the profession of pharmacy, the department shall issue the permit. A permit may not be issued unless a licensed pharmacist is designated to undertake the professional supervision of the compounding and dispensing of all drugs dispensed by the pharmacy. The licensed pharmacist shall be responsible for maintaining all drug records and for providing for the security of the area in the facility in which the compounding, storing, and dispensing of medicinal drugs occurs. The permittee shall notify the department within 10 days after any change of the licensed pharmacist responsible for such duties. Each permittee that employs or otherwise uses registered pharmacy technicians shall have a written policy and procedures manual specifying those duties, tasks, and functions that a registered pharmacy technician is allowed to perform.

Internet Pharmacy Permits

- Any person desiring a permit to operate an Internet pharmacy shall apply to the department for an Internet pharmacy permit. If the board certifies that the application complies with the applicable laws and rules

of the board governing the practice of the profession of pharmacy, the department shall issue the permit. A permit may not be issued unless a licensed pharmacist is designated as the prescription department manager for dispensing medicinal drugs to persons in this state. The licensed pharmacist shall be responsible for maintaining all drug records and for providing for the security of the area in the facility in which the compounding, storing, and dispensing of medicinal drugs to persons in this state occurs. The permittee shall notify the department within 30 days after any change of the licensed pharmacist responsible for such duties. A permittee that employs or otherwise uses registered pharmacy technicians shall have a written policy and procedures manual specifying those duties, tasks, and functions that a registered pharmacy technician is allowed to perform.
- An Internet pharmacy must obtain a permit under this section to sell medicinal drugs to persons in this state.
- An Internet pharmacy shall provide pharmacy services at a high level of protection and competence and shall disclose to the board the following specific information:
    - That it maintains at all times a valid, unexpired license, permit, or registration to operate the pharmacy in compliance with the laws of the state in which the dispensing facility is located and from which the medicinal drugs shall be dispensed.
    - The location, names, and titles of all principal corporate officers and the pharmacist who serves as the prescription department manager for dispensing medicinal drugs to persons in this state. This disclosure shall be made within 30 days after any change of location, principal corporate officer, or pharmacist serving as the prescription department manager for dispensing medicinal drugs to persons in this state.
    - That it complies with all lawful directions and requests for information from the regulatory or

licensing agency of all states in which it is licensed as well as with all requests for information made by the board pursuant to this section. It shall respond directly to all communications from the board concerning emergency circumstances arising from errors in the dispensing of medicinal drugs to persons in this state.
- That it maintains its records of medicinal drugs dispensed to patients in this state so that the records are readily retrievable from the other business records of the pharmacy and from the records of other medicinal drugs dispensed.
- That during its regular hours of operation but not less than 6 days per week, for a minimum of 40 hours per week, a toll-free telephone service shall be provided to facilitate communication between patients in this state and a pharmacist at the pharmacy who has access to the patient's records. This toll-free number must be disclosed on the label affixed to each container of dispensed medicinal drugs.
- Notwithstanding s. 465.003(10), for purposes of this section, the Internet pharmacy and the pharmacist designated by the Internet pharmacy as the prescription department manager or the equivalent must be licensed in the state of location in order to dispense into this state.

Pharmacies; General Requirements
- Must be at least 18 years of age to be issued a pharmacy permit and be fingerprinted. Everyone with at least a 5% ownership interest must also be fingerprinted. Background checks will be done annually.
- Must have written policies and procedures for preventing controlled substance dispensing based on fraudulent representations or invalid practitioner-patient relationships.

- Notify the board within 10 days after any change in prescription department manager or consultant pharmacist of record.
- A registered pharmacist may not serve as the prescription department manager in more than one location unless approved by the board.
- The prescription department manager must notify the board of any theft or significant loss of any controlled substances within 1 business day after discovery of the theft or loss.
- All required records documenting prescription drug distributions shall be readily available or immediately retrievable during an inspection by the department.
- The records must be maintained for 4 years after the creation or receipt of the record, whichever is later.
- Permits issued by the department are not transferable.

Pharmacy Permittee; Disciplinary Action
- The department or the board may revoke or suspend the permit of any pharmacy permittee, and may fine, place on probation, or otherwise discipline any pharmacy permittee if the permittee, or any affiliated person, partner, officer, director, or agent of the permittee, including a person fingerprinted under s. 465.022(3), has:
    o Obtained a permit by misrepresentation or fraud or through an error of the department or the board;
    o Attempted to procure, or has procured, a permit for any other person by making, or causing to be made, any false representation;
    o Violated any of the requirements of this chapter or any of the rules of the Board of Pharmacy; of chapter 499, known as the "Florida Drug and Cosmetic Act"; of 21 U.S.C. ss. 301-392, known as the "Federal Food, Drug, and Cosmetic Act"; of 21 U.S.C. ss. 821 et seq., known as the Comprehensive

> Drug Abuse Prevention and Control Act; or of chapter 893;
> - Been convicted or found guilty, regardless of adjudication, of a felony or any other crime involving moral turpitude in any of the courts of this state, of any other state, or of the United States;
> - Been convicted or disciplined by a regulatory agency of the Federal Government or a regulatory agency of another state for any offense that would constitute a violation of this chapter;
> - Been convicted of, or entered a plea of guilty or nolo contendere to, regardless of adjudication, a crime in any jurisdiction which relates to the practice of, or the ability to practice, the profession of pharmacy;
> - Been convicted of, or entered a plea of guilty or nolo contendere to, regardless of adjudication, a crime in any jurisdiction which relates to health care fraud; or
> - Dispensed any medicinal drug based upon a communication that purports to be a prescription as defined by s. 465.003(14) or s. 893.02 when the pharmacist knows or has reason to believe that the purported prescription is not based upon a valid practitioner-patient relationship that includes a documented patient evaluation, including history and a physical examination adequate to establish the diagnosis for which any drug is prescribed and any other requirement established by board rule under chapter 458, chapter 459, chapter 461, chapter 463, chapter 464, or chapter 466.

- If a pharmacy permit is revoked or suspended, the owner, manager, or proprietor shall cease to operate the establishment as a pharmacy as of the effective date of such suspension or revocation. In the event of such revocation or suspension, the owner, manager, or proprietor shall remove from the premises all signs and symbols identifying the premises as a pharmacy. The period of such suspension shall be prescribed by the Board of Pharmacy, but in no case shall it exceed 1 year. In the event that the permit is revoked, the person owning or operating the establishment shall not be entitled to make application for a permit to operate a pharmacy for a period of 1 year from the date of such revocation. Upon the effective date of such revocation, the permittee shall advise the Board of Pharmacy of the disposition of the medicinal drugs located on the premises. Such disposition shall be subject to continuing supervision and approval by the Board of Pharmacy.

Automated Pharmacy Systems Used By Long-term Care Facilities, Hospices, or State Correctional Institutions

- A pharmacy may provide pharmacy services to a long-term care facility or hospice or a state correctional institution through the use of an automated pharmacy system that need not be located at the same location as the pharmacy.
- Medicinal drugs stored in bulk or unit of use in an automated pharmacy system servicing a long-term care facility, hospice, or correctional institution are part of the inventory of the pharmacy providing pharmacy services to that facility, hospice, or institution, and drugs delivered by the automated pharmacy system are considered to have been dispensed by that pharmacy.
- The operation of an automated pharmacy system must be under the supervision of a Florida-licensed pharmacist. To qualify as a supervisor for an automated pharmacy system, the pharmacist need not be physically present at the site of the automated pharmacy system and may supervise the system electronically. The Florida-licensed pharmacist shall be required to develop and implement

policies and procedures designed to verify that the medicinal drugs delivered by the automated dispensing system are accurate and valid and that the machine is properly restocked.
- Labeling requirements that permit the use of unit-dose medications if the facility, hospice, or institution maintains medication-administration records that include directions for use of the medication and the automated pharmacy system identifies:
    - The dispensing pharmacy;
    - The prescription number;
    - The name of the patient; and
    - The name of the prescribing practitioner.

Promoting Sale of Certain Drugs Prohibited
- No pharmacist, owner, or employee of a retail drug establishment shall use any communication media to promote or advertise the use or sale of any controlled substances.
- This section shall not prohibit the advertising of any medicinal drugs, other than those controlled, or any patent or proprietary preparation, provided the advertising is not false, misleading, or deceptive.

Substitution of Drugs
- A pharmacist who receives a prescription for a brand name drug shall, unless requested otherwise by the purchaser, substitute a less expensive, generically equivalent drug product
- Prescriber must write the words "MEDICALLY NECESSARY" in his or her own handwriting on the face of the prescription if they want the brand name product
- Must inform patient of substitution and they may refuse the substitution
- Each pharmacist shall maintain a record of any substitution of a generically equivalent drug product for a prescribed brand name drug as provided in this section.

- Must display in a prominent place that is in clear and unobstructed public view, at or near the place where prescriptions are dispensed, a sign in block letters not less than 1 inch in height which shall read: "CONSULT YOUR PHARMACIST CONCERNING THE AVAILABILITY OF A LESS EXPENSIVE GENERICALLY EQUIVALENT DRUG AND THE REQUIREMENTS OF FLORIDA LAW."

Expiration Date of Medicinal Drugs; Display; Related Use and Storage Instructions

- The manufacturer, repackager, or other distributor of any medicinal drug shall display the expiration date of each drug in a readable fashion on the container and on its packaging. The term "readable" means conspicuous and bold.
- Each pharmacist for a community pharmacy dispensing medicinal drugs and each practitioner dispensing medicinal drugs on an outpatient basis shall display on the outside of the container of each medicinal drug dispensed, or in other written form delivered to the purchaser:
    - The expiration date when provided by the manufacturer, repackager, or other distributor of the drug; or
    - An earlier beyond-use date for expiration, which may be up to 1 year after the date of dispensing.

Filling of Certain Prescriptions

Nothing contained in this chapter shall be construed to prohibit a pharmacist licensed in this state from filling or refilling a valid prescription which is on file in a pharmacy located in this state or in another state and has been transferred from one pharmacy to another by any means, including any electronic means, under the following conditions:

- Prior to dispensing any transferred prescription, the dispensing pharmacist must, either verbally or by any electronic means, do all of the following:

- Advise the patient that the prescription on file at the other pharmacy must be canceled before it may be filled or refilled.
- Determine that the prescription is valid and on file at the other pharmacy and that the prescription may be filled or refilled, as requested, in accordance with the prescriber's intent expressed on the prescription.
- Notify the pharmacist or pharmacy where the prescription is on file that the prescription must be canceled.
- Record in writing, or by any electronic means, the prescription order, the name of the pharmacy at which the prescription was on file, the prescription number, the name of the drug and the original amount dispensed, the date of original dispensing, and the number of remaining authorized refills.
- Obtain the consent of the prescriber to the refilling of the prescription when the prescription, in the dispensing pharmacist's professional judgment, so requires. Any interference with the professional judgment of the dispensing pharmacist by any pharmacist or pharmacy permittee, or its agents or employees, shall be grounds for discipline.

- Upon receipt of a prescription transfer request, if the pharmacist is satisfied in her or his professional judgment that the request is valid, or if the request has been validated by any electronic means, the pharmacist or pharmacy must do all of the following:
  - Transfer the information required accurately and completely.
  - Record on the prescription, or by any electronic means, the requesting pharmacy and pharmacist and the date of request.

- - Cancel the prescription on file by electronic means or by recording the word "void" on the prescription record. No further prescription information shall be given or medication dispensed pursuant to the original prescription.
- If a transferred prescription is not dispensed within a reasonable time, the pharmacist shall, by any means, so notify the transferring pharmacy. Such notice shall serve to revalidate the canceled prescription. The pharmacist who has served such notice shall then cancel the prescription.
- In the case of a prescription to be transferred from or to a pharmacy located in another state, it shall be the responsibility of the pharmacist or pharmacy located in the State of Florida to verify, whether by electronic means or otherwise, that the person or entity involved in the transfer is a licensed pharmacist or pharmacy in the other state.
- Electronic transfers of prescriptions are permitted regardless of whether the transferor or transferee pharmacy is open for business.
- The transfer of a prescription for medicinal drugs listed in Schedules III, IV, and V for the purpose of refill dispensing is permissible, subject to the requirements of this section and federal law. Compliance with federal law shall be deemed compliance with the requirements of this section.

Centralized Prescription Filling
- A pharmacy licensed under this chapter may perform centralized prescription filling for another pharmacy, provided that the pharmacies have the same owner or have a written contract specifying the services to be provided by each pharmacy.
- The filling, delivery, and return of a prescription by one pharmacy for another pursuant to this section shall not

be construed as the filling of a transferred prescription or as a wholesale distribution.

Common Database
- If a prescription is in a common database then dispensing the prescription does not constitute a transfer

Emergency Prescription Refill
- May dispense a one-time emergency refill of up to a 72-hour supply if unable to obtain refill authorization
- If there is an emergency order or proclamation of a state of emergency declared by the Governor, in which the executive order may authorize the pharmacist to dispense up to a 30-day supply, providing that:
    - Not for a Schedule II
    - Medication is essential to the maintenance of life or to the continuation of therapy in a chronic condition
    - Interruption of therapy might reasonably produce undesirable health consequences or may cause physical or mental discomfort
    - The dispensing pharmacist creates a written order containing all of the prescription information required and signs that order
    - The dispensing pharmacist notifies the prescriber of the emergency dispensing within a reasonable time after such dispensing

Dispensing Practitioner
- A person may not dispense medicinal drugs unless licensed as a pharmacist or otherwise authorized under this chapter to do so, except that a practitioner authorized by law to prescribe drugs may dispense such drugs to her or his patients in the regular course of her or his practice in compliance with this section.
- A practitioner registered under this section may not dispense a controlled substance listed in Schedule II or

Schedule III as provided in s. 893.03. This paragraph does not apply to:
- The dispensing of complimentary packages of medicinal drugs which are labeled as a drug sample or complimentary drug as defined in s. 499.028 to the practitioner's own patients in the regular course of her or his practice without the payment of a fee or remuneration of any kind, whether direct or indirect.
- The dispensing of controlled substances in the health care system of the Department of Corrections.
- The dispensing of a controlled substance listed in Schedule II or Schedule III in connection with the performance of a surgical procedure. The amount dispensed pursuant to the subparagraph may not exceed a 14-day supply. This exception does not allow for the dispensing of a controlled substance listed in Schedule II or Schedule III more than 14 days after the performance of the surgical procedure. For purposes of this subparagraph, the term "surgical procedure" means any procedure in any setting which involves, or reasonably should involve:
    - Perioperative medication and sedation that allows the patient to tolerate unpleasant procedures while maintaining adequate cardiorespiratory function and the ability to respond purposefully to verbal or tactile stimulation and makes intra- and postoperative monitoring necessary; or
    - The use of general anesthesia or major conduction anesthesia and preoperative sedation.
- The dispensing of a controlled substance listed in Schedule II or Schedule III pursuant to an approved clinical trial. For purposes of this

subparagraph, the term "approved clinical trial" means a clinical research study or clinical investigation that, in whole or in part, is state or federally funded or is conducted under an investigational new drug application that is reviewed by the United States Food and Drug Administration.
- o The dispensing of methadone in a facility licensed under s. 397.427 where medication-assisted treatment for opiate addiction is provided.
- o The dispensing of a controlled substance listed in Schedule II or Schedule III to a patient of a facility licensed under part IV of chapter 400.
- A practitioner who dispenses medicinal drugs for human consumption for fee or remuneration of any kind, whether direct or indirect, must:
  - o Register with her or his professional licensing board as a dispensing practitioner and pay a fee not to exceed $100 at the time of such registration and upon each renewal of her or his license. Each appropriate board shall establish such fee by rule.
  - o Comply with and be subject to all laws and rules applicable to pharmacists and pharmacies, including, but not limited to, this chapter and chapters 499 and 893 and all federal laws and federal regulations.
  - o Before dispensing any drug, give the patient a written prescription and orally or in writing advise the patient that the prescription may be filled in the practitioner's office or at any pharmacy.
- The department shall inspect any facility where a practitioner dispenses medicinal drugs pursuant to subsection (2) in the same manner and with the same frequency as it inspects pharmacies for the purpose of determining whether the practitioner is in compliance

- with all statutes and rules applicable to her or his dispensing practice.
- The registration of any practitioner who has been found by her or his respective board to have dispensed medicinal drugs in violation of this chapter shall be subject to suspension or revocation.
- A practitioner who confines her or his activities to the dispensing of complimentary packages of medicinal drugs to the practitioner's own patients in the regular course of her or his practice, without the payment of fee or remuneration of any kind, whether direct or indirect, and who herself or himself dispenses such drugs is not required to register pursuant to this section. The practitioner must dispense such drugs in the manufacturer's labeled package with the practitioner's name, patient's name, and date dispensed, or, if such drugs are not dispensed in the manufacturer's labeled package, they must be dispensed in a container which bears the following information:
    - Practitioner's name;
    - Patient's name;
    - Date dispensed;
    - Name and strength of drug; and
    - Directions for use.

Dispensing of Medicinal Drugs Pursuant to Facsimile of Prescription

- May dispense medicinal drugs including controlled substances based on reception of an electronic facsimile of the original prescription if:
    - The facsimile system making the transmission provides the pharmacy receiving the transmission with audio communication via telephonic, electronic, or similar means with the person presenting the prescription.

- At the time of the delivery of the medicinal drugs, the pharmacy has in its possession the original prescription for the medicinal drug involved.
- The recipient of the prescription shall sign a log and shall indicate the name and address of both the recipient and the patient for whom the medicinal drug was prescribed.

Rebates Prohibited

It is unlawful for any person to pay or receive any commission, bonus, kickback, or rebate or engage in any split-fee arrangement in any form whatsoever with any physician, surgeon, organization, agency, or person, either directly or indirectly, for patients referred to a registered pharmacy.

Pharmacist's Order for Medicinal Drugs

- There is hereby created a committee composed of two members of the Board of Medicine licensed under chapter 458 chosen by said board, one member of the Board of Osteopathic Medicine licensed under chapter 459 chosen by said board, three members of the Board of Pharmacy licensed under this chapter and chosen by said board, and one additional person with a background in health care or pharmacology chosen by the committee. The committee shall establish a formulary of medicinal drug products and dispensing procedures which shall be used by a pharmacist when ordering and dispensing such drug products to the public. Dispensing procedures may include matters related to reception of patient, description of his or her condition, patient interview, patient physician referral, product selection, and dispensing and use limitations. In developing the formulary of medicinal drug products, the committee may include products falling within the following categories:
    - Any medicinal drug of single or multiple active ingredients in any strengths when such active

- ingredients have been approved individually or in combination for over-the-counter sale by the United States Food and Drug Administration.
  - Any medicinal drug recommended by the United States Food and Drug Administration Advisory Panel for transfer to over-the-counter status pending approval by the United States Food and Drug Administration.
  - Any medicinal drug containing any antihistamine or decongestant as a single active ingredient or in combination.
  - Any medicinal drug containing fluoride in any strength.
  - Any medicinal drug containing lindane in any strength.
  - Any over-the-counter proprietary drug under federal law that has been approved for reimbursement by the Florida Medicaid Program.
  - Any topical anti-infectives excluding eye and ear topical anti-infectives.

However, any drug which is sold as an over-the-counter proprietary drug under federal law shall not be included in the formulary or otherwise affected by this section.

- The Board of Pharmacy, the Board of Medicine, and the Board of Osteopathic Medicine shall adopt by rule a formulary of medicinal drugs and dispensing procedures as established by the committee. A pharmacist may order and dispense a product from the formulary pursuant to the established dispensing procedure, as adopted by the boards, for each drug in conjunction with its inclusion in the formulary. Any drug product ordered by a pharmacist shall be selected and dispensed only by the pharmacist so ordering, and said order shall not be refilled, nor shall another medicinal drug be ordered for the same condition unless such act is consistent with dispensing procedures established by the committee. Appropriate referral to another health care provider is indicated

under such circumstances. On each occasion of such dispensing, the pharmacist shall create and maintain a prescription record in the form required by law.
- Affixed to the container containing a medicinal drug dispensed pursuant to this section shall be a label bearing the following information:
    - The name of the pharmacist ordering the medication.
    - The name and address of the pharmacy from which the medication was dispensed.
    - The date of dispensing.
    - The order number or other identification adequate to readily identify the order.
    - The name of the patient for whom the medicinal drug was ordered.
    - The directions for use of the medicinal drug ordered.
    - A clear, concise statement that the order may not be refilled.

Medicaid Audits of Pharmacies
- Notwithstanding any other law, when an audit of the Medicaid-related records of a pharmacy licensed under chapter 465 is conducted, such audit must be conducted as provided in this section.
    - The agency conducting the audit must give the pharmacist at least 1 week's prior notice of the initial audit for each audit cycle.
    - An audit must be conducted by a pharmacist licensed in this state.
    - Any clerical or recordkeeping error, such as a typographical error, scrivener's error, or computer error regarding a document or record required under the Medicaid program does not constitute a willful violation and is not subject to criminal penalties without proof of intent to commit fraud.

- A pharmacist may use the physician's record or other order for drugs or medicinal supplies written or transmitted by any means of communication for purposes of validating the pharmacy record with respect to orders or refills of a legend or narcotic drug.
- A finding of an overpayment or underpayment must be based on the actual overpayment or underpayment and may not be a projection based on the number of patients served having a similar diagnosis or on the number of similar orders or refills for similar drugs.
- Each pharmacy shall be audited under the same standards and parameters.
- A pharmacist must be allowed at least 10 days in which to produce documentation to address any discrepancy found during an audit.
- The period covered by an audit may not exceed 1 calendar year.
- An audit may not be scheduled during the first 5 days of any month due to the high volume of prescriptions filled during that time.
- The audit report must be delivered to the pharmacist within 90 days after conclusion of the audit. A final audit report shall be delivered to the pharmacist within 6 months after receipt of the preliminary audit report or final appeal, whichever is later.

- The Agency for Health Care Administration shall establish a process under which a pharmacist may obtain a preliminary review of an audit report and may appeal an unfavorable audit report without the necessity of obtaining legal counsel. The preliminary review and appeal may be conducted by an ad hoc peer review panel, appointed by the agency, which consists of pharmacists who maintain an active practice. If, following the preliminary review, the agency or review panel finds that an unfavorable audit report is unsubstantiated, the agency shall dismiss the audit report without the necessity of any further proceedings.

Administration of Influenza Virus Immunizations

- Pharmacists may administer influenza virus immunizations to adults within the framework of an established protocol under a supervisory practitioner.
- A pharmacist may not enter into a protocol unless he or she maintains at least $200,000 of professional liability insurance and has completed training in influenza virus immunizations as provided in this section.
- Maintain records for a minimum of 5 years.
- Any pharmacist seeking to administer influenza virus immunizations to adults under this section must be certified to administer influenza virus immunizations pursuant to a certification program approved by the Board of Pharmacy in consultation with the Board of Medicine and the Board of Osteopathic Medicine. The certification program shall, at a minimum, require that the pharmacist attend at least 20 hours of continuing education classes approved by the board. The program shall have a curriculum of instruction concerning the safe and effective administration of influenza virus immunizations, including, but not limited to, potential allergic reactions to influenza virus immunizations.
- The written protocol between the pharmacist and supervising physician must include particular terms and conditions imposed by the supervising physician upon the pharmacist relating to the administration of influenza virus immunizations by the pharmacist. The written protocol shall include, at a minimum, specific categories and conditions among patients for whom the supervising physician authorizes the pharmacist to administer influenza virus immunizations. The terms, scope, and conditions set forth in the written protocol between the pharmacist and the supervising physician must be

appropriate to the pharmacist's training and certification for immunization. Pharmacists who have been delegated the authority to administer influenza virus immunizations by the supervising physician shall provide evidence of current certification by the Board of Pharmacy to the supervising physician. Supervising physicians shall review the administration of influenza virus immunizations by the pharmacists under such physician's supervision pursuant to the written protocol, and this review shall take place as outlined in the written protocol. The process and schedule for the review shall be outlined in the written protocol between the pharmacist and the supervising physician.
- The pharmacist shall submit to the Board of Pharmacy a copy of his or her protocol or written agreement to administer influenza virus immunizations.

Section Eight: Florida Law Chapter 64B16-25

Probable Cause Panel
- Determines whether probable cause exists to believe that a violation of the chapters or rules has occurred
- Composed of two persons appointed by the chairman of the Board
    - Current board member
    - Licensed pharmacist that is a former or current board member

Initial License Fees
- Pharmacist license shall be $190 plus a $5 unlicensed activity fee
- Consultant pharmacist license shall be $50 plus a $5 unlicensed activity fee
- Nuclear pharmacist license shall be $50 plus a $5 unlicensed activity fee
- Registered pharmacy technician shall be $50 plus a $5 unlicensed activity fee

Active License Renewal Fees
- Biennial license renewal fee for an active pharmacist license shall be $200 plus a $5 unlicensed activity fee
- Biennial license renewal fee for a consultant pharmacist active license shall be $100 plus a $5 unlicensed activity fee
- Biennial license renewal fee for a nuclear pharmacist active license shall be $100 plus a $5 unlicensed activity fee
- Biennial registration renewal fee for a registered pharmacy technician shall be $50 plus $5 unlicensed activity fee

Inactive License Election
- A pharmacist licensee, consultant pharmacist licensee, nuclear pharmacist licensee, and registered pharmacy technician may elect to:
    - Place the license on inactive status – submit written request to the board and pay fee
    - Continue the license on inactive status – submit written request to the board and pay fee
    - Changing from inactive to active – must have the required CE from each biennium the license was inactive and pay fees

Retired License Election
- Place the license on retired status – submit written request to the board and pay fee
- Reactivating a retired license – must have all the required CE from each biennium the license was retired and pay all fees
    - If inactive for less than 5 years – must pass the MPJE
    - If inactive for 5 or more years – must pass the NAPLEX and MPJE

Delinquent License Reversion
- An active or inactive license that is not renewed by midnight of the expiration date of the license shall automatically revert to delinquent status
- Reinstate a pharmacist delinquent license = complete all CE requirements and pay fees
- Reinstate a delinquent consultant pharmacist license = pay fees
- Reinstate a delinquent nuclear pharmacist license = pay fees
- Reinstate a delinquent registered pharmacy technician = complete all CE requirements and pay fees
- A license in delinquent status that is not renewed prior to midnight of the expiration date of the current licensure

cycle shall be rendered null and must apply for a new license

CE for Pharmacist
Minimum of 30 hours required within the 24 months prior to renewal of pharmacist licensure
The following conditions shall apply:
- Upon a licensee's first renewal of licensure – must complete 1 hour of board approved CE which includes the topics of Human Immunodeficiency Virus and Acquired Immune Deficiency Syndrome includes information on the State of Florida law on HIV/AIDS and its impact on testing, reporting, the offering of HIV testing to pregnant women, and partner notification
- No CE required if initial license was issued less than 12 months prior to the expiration date of the license
- 15 hours of CE required if initial renewal occurs 12 months or more after the initial licensure
- 2 hours of CE approved by the Board on medication errors required prior to license renewal
- 5 hours of CE obtained by attending one full day or 8 hours of a board meeting at which disciplinary hearings are conducted by the Board of Pharmacy in compliance with the following:
    - Sign in with the Executive Director or designee of the Board before the meeting day begins
    - Remain in continuous attendance
    - Cannot receive continuing education credit for attendance at a board meeting if required to appear before the board; and
    - Maximum continuing education hours allowable per biennium shall be ten (10)
- Up to 5 hours per biennium may be fulfilled by the performance of volunteer services to the indigent. One hour credit shall be given for each two hours volunteered in the 24 months prior to the expiration date of the license. Must be approved by the Board first.

- 5 hours of CE for each semester hour completed of a post professional degree programs provided by accredited colleges or schools of pharmacy
- Volunteer expert witness receive 5 CE hours per each case reviewed up to a max of 10 hours per biennium
- CE presenter earns 1 credit hour for each hour presented – but not multiple presentations of the same thing
- All programs approved by the ACPE for CE are allowed by the Board but any course necessary to meet the continuing education requirement for HIV/AIDS, medication errors, or consultant pharmacist license renewal shall be Board approved
- CE earned by a non-resident pharmacist in another state that is approved by the board in that state will qualify for CE in this state
- Minimum of 10 CE hours must be live

CE for a Consultant Pharmacist

- Minimum of 24 hours of CE required for license renewal in addition to the 30 hours required to renew a pharmacist license
- No CE required if initial renewal occurs less than 12 months after the initial licensure
- 12 hours of consultant CE required if the initial renewal occurs 12 months or more after the initial licensure

CE for a Nuclear Pharmacist

- Minimum of 24 hours of CE required for license renewal in addition to the 30 hours required to renew a pharmacist license
- No CE required if initial renewal occurs less than 12 months after the initial licensure
- 12 hours of nuclear pharmacy CE required if the initial renewal occurs 12 months or more after the initial licensure
- All ACPE approved nuclear pharmacist CE are approved by the Board for nuclear pharmacist CE

CE for a Registered Pharmacy Technician
- 20 hours of CE required prior to license renewal
- Upon first renewal, one hour of board approved CE in HIV/AIDS must be completed
- No CE required if initial renewal occurs less than 12 months after the initial licensure
- 12 hours of CE required if the initial renewal occurs 12 months or more after the initial licensure
- 2 hours of CE on medication errors must be completed prior to license renewal
- 4 of the 20 hours must be obtained live

Influenza Immunization Certification Program
- Certification program for pharmacist administration of influenza immunizations
- Minimum of 20 hours of study that includes a successful demonstration of competency in the administration technique and a cognitive examination

Exemptions for Members of the Armed Forces; Spouses
- Active duty pharmacist or registered pharmacy technician in good standing is exempt from all license renewal provisions so long as the licensee is on active duty with the Armed Forces and for a period of six months after discharge so long as the licensee is not engaged in the practice of pharmacy in the private sector for profit
- A pharmacist or registered pharmacy technician who is a spouse of a member of the Armed Forces of the United States and who was caused to be absent from the State of Florida because of the spouse's duties with the Armed Forces shall be exempt from all license renewal provisions

Examination Requirement
- North American Pharmacist Licensure Examination (NAPLEX)
- Multistate Pharmacy Jurisprudence Examination – Florida Version

Licensure by Examination; Application
- Must be at least 18 years of age and receive a degree from an ACPE accredited school of pharmacy
- Make application to the board and pay fees
- Submit proof of having met the following requirements:
    - Completion of an internship program provided by either an accredited school or college of pharmacy or a state board of pharmacy or jointly by both
    - Completion of a board approved course not less than 2 hours on medication errors that covers the study of root-cause analysis, error reduction and prevention, and patient safety. For those applicants who apply within one year following receipt of their pharmacy degree, completed academic course work on medication errors will be accepted by the Board as an educational course under this section, provided such course work is no less than 2 contact hours and that it covers the study of root-cause analysis, error reduction and prevention, and patient safety, as evidenced by a letter attesting to subject matter covered from the Dean of the University.
- Must reapply if all requirements for licensure are not met within one year of the receipt of the application
- Passing examination scores only good for 3 years

Licensure by Examination; Foreign Pharmacy Graduates
- In order for a foreign pharmacy graduate to be admitted to the professional licensure examination, the applicant

must be a graduate of a four year undergraduate pharmacy program at a school or college outside the United States and have completed an internship program approved by the Board
- Apply to the board and pay fees
- Successfully pass the foreign pharmacy graduate equivalency examination with a minimum score of 75%
- Pass the Test of English as a Foreign Language (TOEFL)
- Complete 2080 hours of supervised work activity, of which a minimum of 500 hours must be completed within the State of Florida and must pass the Foreign Pharmacy Graduate Equivalency Examination first
- Completion of a Board approved course not less than 2 hours on medication errors that covers the study of root-cause analysis, error reduction and prevention, and patient safety. For applicants who apply within one year following receipt of their pharmacy degree, completed academic course work on medication errors will be accepted by the Board as an educational course under this section, provided such course work is no less than 2 contact hours and that it covers the study of root-cause analysis, error reduction and prevention, and patient safety as evidence by a letter attesting to subject matter covered from the Dean of the University.

Pharmacy Intern Registration Internship Requirements (U.S. Pharmacy Students/Graduates)

- A U.S. pharmacy student or graduate is required to be registered with the Department of Health as an intern before being employed as an intern in a pharmacy in Florida
- Apply to the board and pay fees
- Submit proof of:
    - Enrollment in an intern program at a college or school of pharmacy accredited by the Accreditation Council of Pharmaceutical Education (ACPE); or

- Graduation from a college or school of pharmacy accredited by the ACPE
- No intern shall perform any acts relating to the filing, compounding, or dispensing of medicinal drugs unless it is done under the direct and immediate personal supervision of a person actively licensed to practice pharmacy in this state
- No pharmacist may be responsible for the supervision of more than one intern at any one time
- Any applicant submitting for the purpose of qualifying for licensure by examination must show in addition to successful completion of the internship:
    - Approval of the program by a state board of pharmacy; and
    - Sufficient hours to total 2080 hours; or
    - Licensure in another state and work performed as a pharmacist for a sufficient number of hours to total 2080 hours when combined with the internship hours
- All internship hours may be obtained prior to the applicant's graduation
- Maximum of 50 hours per week prior to the applicant's graduation or 60 hours per week after an applicant's graduation
- Proof of current licensure in another state and work as a pharmacist for up to 2080 hours may substitute for all or part of the internship requirement.
- Governmental and private radiopharmacy internship programs shall not apply to the pharmacy internship

Pharmacy Intern Registration and Internship Requirements (Foreign Pharmacy Graduates)

- A foreign pharmacy graduate is required to be registered with the Department of Health as an intern before being employed as an intern in a pharmacy in Florida
- Make application to the board

- An applicant for foreign pharmacy graduate intern registration in Florida must submit proof of:
    - Eligibility by the Foreign Pharmacy Graduate Equivalency Committee to sit for the Foreign Pharmacy Graduate Equivalency Examination, or
    - A passing score on the Foreign Pharmacy Graduate Equivalency Examination to be considered a graduate of an accredited college or school of pharmacy
- No intern shall perform any acts relating to the filling, compounding, or dispensing of medicinal drugs unless it is done under the direct and immediate personal supervision of a person actively licensed to practice pharmacy in this state.
- No pharmacist may be responsible for the supervision of more than one intern at any one time.
- In the event a program meets all the requirements, except for prior approval by the Florida Board of Pharmacy, any applicant submitting it for the purpose of qualifying for licensure by examination must show in addition to successful completion of the internship:
    - Approval of the program by a state board of pharmacy; and
    - Sufficient hours to total 1580 hours; or
    - Licensure in another state and work performed as a pharmacist for a sufficient number of hours to total 1580 hours when combined with the internship hours
- All internship hours may be obtained prior to the applicant's graduation
- Proof of completion of an internship program shall consist of a certification that the applicant has completed the program. If additional hours are required to total 2080 hours, satisfactory proof of the additional hours shall be constituted by the program's certification of completion of the additional hours.

- Maximum of 50 hours per week prior to the applicant's graduation or 60 hours per week after an applicant's graduation
- Proof of current licensure in another state and work as a pharmacist for up to 1580 hours may substitute for all or part of the internship hours requirement
- All foreign pharmacy graduates must complete 500 hours of supervised work activity within the state of Florida. Must pass Foreign Pharmacy Graduate Equivalency Exam before beginning these hours

Licensure by Endorsement

- Must be at least 18 years of age and receive a pharmacy degree from an ACPE accredited school/college
- Apply to the board and pay fees
- Applicant must submit satisfactory proof that one of the following requirements has been met:
    - Two (2) years of active practice within the immediately preceding five (5) years. Also must have 30 hours of CE obtained in the two calendar years immediately preceding application; OR
    - Successful completion of an internship meeting the requirements of Section 465.007(1)(c), F.S., within the immediately preceding two (2) years
- 2 hours of CE on medication errors that covers the study of root-cause analysis, error reduction and prevention, and patient safety
- Foreign graduates must complete the requirements of Rule 64B16-26.2031 prior to certification for the examination
- All requirements for licensure by endorsement must be met within one (1) year of the receipt of the application. Applicants failing to meet this requirement must reapply.
- Applicants applying under the provisions of Section 465.0075, F.S., must have obtained a passing score on the licensure examination as described in subsection 64B16-26.200(1), F.A.C.

- Applicants applying under the provisions of Section 465.0075, F.S., shall cause the National Association of Boards of Pharmacy, or other similar organization to issue a Transfer of Pharmaceutical Licensure certificate showing examination date, examination results, states of licensure, disciplinary actions, and licensure status.
- Applicants deemed qualified for licensure by endorsement shall be required to complete the Multistate Pharmacy Jurisprudence Examination – Florida Version. Passing scores on this examination may be used upon reapplication only if the examination was completed within three (3) years of the reapplication.

Consultant Pharmacist Licensure
- No person shall serve as consultant pharmacist unless that person holds a license as a consultant pharmacist
- Apply to the board and pay fees
- In order to be licensed as a consultant pharmacist, a person must meet the following requirements:
    - Hold a license as a pharmacist which is active and in good standing
    - Successfully complete a consultant pharmacist course of no fewer than twelve (12) hours, sponsored by an accredited college of pharmacy located within the State of Florida, and approved by the Florida Board of Pharmacy Tripartite Continuing Education Committee. The course shall be instructionally designed to include a cognitive test on which the applicant must score a passing grade for certification of successful completion of the course.
    - Successfully complete a period of assessment and evaluation under the supervision of a preceptor within one (1) year of completion of the course. This period of assessment and evaluation shall be completed over no more than three (3) consecutive months and shall include at least 40

hours of training in the following practice areas, 60% of which shall occur on-site at an institution that holds a pharmacy permit. The training shall include a minimum of 40 Hours in maximum of three months.
- In order to act as a preceptor, a person shall:
    - Be a consultant pharmacist of record at an institutional pharmacy which is required to have a consultant pharmacist.
    - Have a minimum of one (1) year of experience as a consultant pharmacist of record.
    - Maintain all pharmacist licenses in good standing with the Board
    - Not act as a preceptor to more than two (2) applicants at the same time.
- Upon completion of the requirements set forth above, the applicant's preceptor shall confirm that the applicant's assessment and evaluation have met the requirements and that the applicant has successfully completed all required assignments under the preceptor's guidance and supervision.
- After licensure a consultant pharmacist's license shall be renewed biennially upon payment of the fee, and upon completing twenty-four (24) hours of board approved continuing education.
- The number of hours earned in recertification programs by a consultant pharmacist, if applied to the twenty-four (24) hours required for consultant pharmacist license renewal, may not be used toward the thirty (30) hours of continued professional pharmaceutical education credits.

Nuclear Pharmacist Licensure
- A pharmacist licensed to practice pharmacy in this state who performs a radiopharmaceutical service shall, prior to engaging in such specialized practice, be actively licensed as a nuclear pharmacist.

- A pharmacist seeking licensure as a nuclear pharmacist in this state shall submit to the Board of Pharmacy a course outline from an accredited college of pharmacy or other program recognized by the Florida Department of Health and the Florida Board of Pharmacy (a program comparable to those offered by accredited colleges of pharmacy for the training of nuclear pharmacists), and a certificate of training which provides a minimum of 200 clock hours of formal didactic training, which includes:
    - Radiation physics and instrumentation (85 hours)
    - Radiation protection (45 hours)
    - Mathematics pertaining to the use and measurement of radioactivity (20 hours)
    - Radiation biology (20 hours)
    - Radiopharmaceutical chemistry (30 hours)
- Such academic training programs will be submitted to the Board of Pharmacy for approval by an accredited educational institution which operates under the auspices of or in conjunction with an accredited college of pharmacy
- The minimum on-the-job training which shall be included in a radiopharmacy internship is 500 hours of training and experience in the handling of unsealed radioactive material under the supervision of a licensed nuclear pharmacist. The training and experience shall include but shall not be limited to the following:
    - Ordering, receiving and unpackaging in a safe manner, radioactive material, including the performance of related radiation surveys
    - Calibrating dose calibrators, scintillation detectors, and radiation monitoring equipment
    - Calculating, preparing and verifying patient doses, including the proper use of radiation shields
    - Following appropriate internal control procedures to prevent mislabeling

- - Learning emergency procedures to safely handle and contain spilled materials, including related decontamination procedures and surveys
  - Eluting technetium-99m from generator systems, assaying the eluate for technetium-99m and for molybdenum-99 contamination, and processing the eluate with reagent kits to prepare technetium-99m labeled radiopharmaceuticals
  - Clinical practice concepts
- If the didactic and experiential training required in this section have not been completed within the last seven (7) years, the applicant must have been engaged in the lawful practice of nuclear pharmacy in another jurisdiction at least 1080 hours during the last seven (7) years.

CE for Nuclear Pharmacist License Renewal
- 24 hours every 2 years

Subject Matter for Continuing Education to Order and Evaluate Laboratory Tests
- Consultant pharmacists and PharmD's that wish to order and evaluate laboratory tests are required to complete the requirements of a CE course. Successful completion of the course will certify the pharmacist for this practice for two (2) years from date of completion.
- Courses approved under this section shall be at least three (3) hours in duration for initial certification and at least one (1) hour for recertification, and shall cover the following subjects:
  - Requirements for monitoring laboratory values
  - Interpretation of laboratory values
  - Use of laboratory data to monitor and improve drug therapy
  - Legal aspects, restrictions, and requirements for obtaining laboratory studies
  - Use of laboratory data and therapeutic outcomes
  - Documentation of interventions, and

- o Laboratory studies as an element of complete patient care
- A consultant pharmacist may apply the three (3) hour initial certification course and the one (1) hour recertification course toward the continuing education requirement for renewal of a consultant pharmacist license or may apply such continuing education hours toward the continuing education requirement for renewal of a pharmacist license, but may not use the same continuing education hours to satisfy both requirements. A Doctor of Pharmacy who is not a consultant pharmacist may apply the three (3) hour initial certification course and the one (1) hour recertification course toward the continuing education requirement for renewal of a pharmacist license.

Requirements for Pharmacy Technician Registration
- Applicants who are at least 17 years of age may apply to become a registered pharmacy technician.
- Apply to board and pay fees
- Prior to January 1, 2011, a registered pharmacy technician must submit proof of having met one of the following requirements:
    - o Completed a Board approved training course; or
    - o Worked as a registered pharmacy technician for a minimum of 1500 hours under the supervision of a pharmacist; or
    - o Received certification as a pharmacy technician by a certification program accredited by the National Commission for Certifying Agencies
- Applicants applying for registration after January 1, 2011 must submit proof of completion of a Board approved training course

Standards for Approval of Registered Pharmacy Technician Training Programs

- The following programs are approved Registered Pharmacy Technician Training programs:
    - Pharmacy technician training programs accredited, on or before January 1, 2011 by the American Society of Health-System Pharmacists
    - Pharmacy technician training programs at institutions accredited, on or before January 1, 2011 by the Southern Association of Colleges and Schools,
    - Pharmacy technician training programs approved on or before January 1, 2011 by the Florida Commission for Independent Education,
    - Pharmacy technician training programs provided by a branch of the federal armed services on or before January 1, 2011.
    - Pharmacy technician training programs at institutions accredited on or before January 1, 2011 by the Council on Occupational Education.
- All programs not listed above and which are not employer based programs, must:
    - Meet the requirements of and be licensed by the Commission for Independent Education pursuant to Chapter 1005, F.S., or the equivalent licensing authority of another state or be within the public school system of the State of Florida; and:
    - Offer a course of study that includes classroom study and clinical instruction
- Apply directly to the Board of Pharmacy on approved form DH-MQA 1239 "Board of Pharmacy Application for Registered Pharmacy Technician Training Programs,"
- All other training programs must be employer based. Any pharmacy technician training program sponsored by a Florida permitted pharmacy or affiliated group of pharmacies under common ownership, must contain a minimum of 160 hours of training, that extends over a

period not to exceed 6 months; is provided solely to employees of said pharmacy or affiliated group; and has been approved by the Board. An application for approval of a Registered Pharmacy Technician Training Program shall be made on Board of Pharmacy approved form DH-MQA 1239 "Board of Pharmacy Application for Registered Pharmacy Technician Training Programs," effective December 2010. The applicant must attach to the application copy of curriculum, catalog or other course description. All employer based programs must:
- Ensure that self-directed learning experiences, including but not limited to home study, computer programs, internet or web-based courses evaluate participant knowledge at the completion of the learning experience. The evaluation must include a minimum of 100 questions. The participant must achieve a minimum score of 70% on the evaluation to receive the certificate of completion. The evaluation must be graded by the provider.
- Maintain program records for a period not less than three years during which time the records must be available for inspection by the board or department.
- Furnish each participant with an authenticated individual Certificate of Completion.

Pharmacy Interns; Registration; Employment
- Must be registered with the Department of Health as an intern before being employed as an intern in a pharmacy in Florida
- An applicant for pharmacy intern registration must submit proof of:
  - Enrollment in an intern program at an accredited college or school of pharmacy or;
  - Graduation from an accredited college or school of pharmacy and not yet licensed in the state. For purposes of this rule only, any individual who has

been accepted by the Foreign Pharmacy Graduate Examination Commission to sit for the Foreign Pharmacy Graduate Equivalency Examination shall be considered a graduate of an accredited college or school of pharmacy. The internship experience allowed under this provision shall not count toward the 500-hours internship required subsequent to passage of the Foreign Pharmacy Graduate Equivalency Examination
- No intern shall perform any acts relating to the filling, compounding, or dispensing of medicinal drugs unless it is done under the direct and immediate personal supervision of a person actively licensed to practice pharmacy in this state

Tripartite Continuing Education Committee
- Composed of equal representation from the Board of Pharmacy, each College or School of Pharmacy in the State, and practicing pharmacists within the State. The members of the Committee shall be selected by the Board of Pharmacy and shall serve for a period of two years. The chairman of the committee shall be selected by the Chair of the Board.
- Perform the following duties:
    - Review continuing education providers and make recommendations to the Board;
    - Approve continuing education course or program for approved providers or individuals that are non-approved providers for the following:
- Perform auditing and monitoring activities The Tripartite Committee shall perform an audit on each approved continuing education provider 90 days prior to the end of the biennium.

Continuing Education Records Requirements
- Keep for at least two years after the license is renewed

Section Nine: Pharmacy Practice

Display of Current License; Pharmacist, Registered, Intern, and Registered Pharmacy Technician Identification
- Current license of each pharmacist and registered pharmacy technicians must be displayed in the pharmacy and easily read by customers. If employed at a secondary pharmacy, keep a valid wallet license.
- A pharmacist and registered pharmacy intern must be clearly identified by a means such as an identification badge or monogrammed smock showing their name and if they are a pharmacist or a registered pharmacy intern.

Practice of Pharmacy
- A pharmacist or registered pharmacy intern must:
    - Supervise and be responsible for the controlled substance inventory.
    - Receive verbal prescriptions from a practitioner.
    - Interpret and identify prescription contents.
    - Engage in consultation with a practitioner regarding interpretation of the prescription and date in patient profile.
    - Engage in professional communication with practitioners, nurses or other health professionals.
    - Advise or consult with a patient, both as to the prescription and the patient profile record.
- When parenteral and bulk solutions of all sizes are prepared, regardless of the route of administration, the pharmacist must:
    - Interpret and identify all incoming orders.
    - Mix all extemporaneous compounding or be physically present and give direction to the registered pharmacy technician for reconstitution, for addition of additives, or for bulk compounding of the parenteral solution.

- - Physically examine, certify to the accuracy of the final preparation, thereby assuming responsibility for the final preparation.
  - Systemize all records and documentation of processing in such a manner that professional responsibility can be easily traced to a pharmacist.
- Only a pharmacist may make the final check of the completed prescription thereby assuming the complete responsibility for its preparation and accuracy.
- The pharmacist, as an integral aspect of dispensing, shall be directly and immediately available to the patient or the patient's agent for consultation and shall not dispense to a third party. No prescription shall be deemed to be properly dispensed unless the pharmacist is personally available.
- The pharmacist may take a meal break, not to exceed 30 minutes in length, during which the pharmacy department of a permittee shall not be considered closed, under the following conditions:
  - The pharmacist shall be considered present and on duty during any such meal break if a sign has been prominently posted in the pharmacy indicating the specific hours of the day during which meal breaks may be taken by the pharmacist and assuring patients that a pharmacist is available on the premises for consultation upon request during a meal break.
  - The pharmacist shall be considered directly and immediately available to patients during such meal breaks if patients to whom medications are delivered during meal breaks are verbally informed that they may request that a pharmacist contact them at the pharmacist's earliest convenience after the meal break, and if a pharmacist is available on the premises during the meal break for consultation regarding emergency

matters. Only prescriptions with the final certification by the pharmacist may be delivered.
    - The activities of registered pharmacy technicians during such a meal break shall be considered to be under the direct and immediate personal supervision of a pharmacist if the pharmacist is available on the premises during the meal break to respond to questions by the technicians, and if at the end of the meal break the pharmacist certifies all prescriptions prepared by the registered pharmacy technicians during the meal break.
- The delegation of any duties, tasks or functions to registered pharmacy interns and registered pharmacy technicians must be performed subject to a continuing review and ultimate supervision of the pharmacist who instigated the specific task, so that a continuity of supervised activity is present between one pharmacist and one registered pharmacy technician. In every pharmacy, the pharmacist shall retain the professional and personal responsibility for any delegated act performed by registered pharmacy interns and registered pharmacy technicians in the licensee's employ or under the licensee's supervision.

Oral Prescriptions and Copies
- Only a pharmacist or registered pharmacy intern acting under the supervision of a pharmacist may, in the State of Florida, accept an oral prescription of any nature.
- Only a pharmacist or registered pharmacy intern acting under the supervision of a pharmacist may, in the State of Florida, prepare a copy of a prescription or read a prescription to any person for purposes of providing reference concerning treatment of the person or animal for whom the prescription was written, and when said copy is given a notation shall be made upon the

prescription that a copy has been given, the date given, and to whom given.

Conduct Governing Pharmacists and Pharmacy Permittees

- A pharmacist or pharmacy shall be permitted to advertise medicinal drugs other than those controlled substances, and patent and proprietary preparations so long as such advertising is not false, misleading or deceptive.
- No pharmacist, employer or employee of a pharmacy shall maintain a location, other than a pharmacy for which a permit has been issued by the Florida Board of Pharmacy, from which to solicit, accept or dispense prescriptions.
- No pharmacist or pharmacy, or employee or agent thereof, shall enter into or engage in any agreement or arrangement with any physician or other practitioner or nursing home or extended care facility for the payment or acceptance of compensation in any form or type for the recommending of the professional services of either; or enter into a rebate or percentage rental agreement of any kind, whereby in any way a patient's free choice of a pharmacist or pharmacy is or may be limited.
- No pharmacist, employer or employee of a pharmacy may knowingly place in stock of any pharmacy any part of any prescription compounded for, or dispensed to, any customer of any pharmacy and returned by said customer, unless otherwise specified.
- A permit for a community pharmacy may not be issued unless a licensed pharmacist is designated as the prescription department manager responsible for maintaining all drug records, providing for the security of the prescription department and following such other rules as relate to the practice of the profession of pharmacy. The Board shall not register a prescription department manager as the manager of more than one

pharmacy. The Board shall grant an exception to this requirement upon application by the permittee and the prescription department manager showing circumstances such as proximity of permits and limited pharmacist workload that would allow the manager to carry out all duties and responsibilities required of a prescription department manager.

Transfer of Prescriptions
- A pharmacist or registered pharmacy intern acting under the direct personal supervision of a Florida registered pharmacist may transfer a valid prescription which is on file in another pharmacy in this state or any other state. Prior to dispensing, the pharmacist or pharmacy where the prescription is on file shall be notified verbally, or by any electronic means that the former prescription must be voided.
- In processing a transferred prescription, the pharmacist has the option of substituting a generically equivalent product.

Ordering and Evaluation of Laboratory Tests
Those consultant pharmacists and pharmacists holding the Doctor of Pharmacy degree that meet the continuing education requirements, may order and evaluate laboratory tests. Evidence of such training and authorization to perform these tasks shall be furnished to the board, the patient, or the patient's physician upon request.

General Terms and Conditions to Be Followed by a Pharmacist When Ordering and Dispensing Approved Medicinal Drug Products
A pharmacist may order the medicinal drug products, but subject to the following terms and limitations:
- Injectable products shall not be ordered by the pharmacist.

- No oral medicinal drugs shall be ordered by a pharmacist for a pregnant patient or nursing mother.
- In any case of dispensing hereunder, the amount or quantity of drug dispensed shall not exceed a 34-day supply or standard course of treatment unless subject to the specific limitations in this rule. Patients shall be advised that they should seek the advice of an appropriate health care provider if their present condition, symptom, or complaint does not improve upon the completion of the drug regimen.
- The directions for use of all prescribed medicinal drugs shall not exceed the manufacturer's recommended dosage.
- The pharmacist may only perform the acts of ordering and dispensing in a pharmacy which has been issued a permit by the Board of Pharmacy.
- The pharmacist shall create a prescription when ordering and dispensing medicinal drug products which shall be maintained in the prescription files of the pharmacy. The pharmacist shall place the trade or generic name and the quantity dispensed on the prescription label, in addition to all other label requirements.
- The pharmacist shall maintain patient profiles, separate from the prescription order, for all patients for whom the pharmacist orders and dispenses medicinal drug products and shall initial and date each profile entry. Such profiles shall be maintained at the pharmacy wherein the ordering and dispensing originated for a period of two (2) years.
- In the patient profiles, the pharmacist shall record as a minimum the following information if a medicinal drug product is ordered and dispensed.
    - Patient's chief complaint or condition in the patient's own words.
    - A statement regarding the patient's medical history.

- o A statement regarding the patient's current complaint which may include, onset, duration and frequency of the problem.
- o The medicinal drug product ordered and dispensed.
- o The pharmacist ordering and dispensing the medicinal drug product shall initial the profile.
- o The prescription number shall be recorded in the patient's profile.
* A medicinal drug product may be ordered, and dispensed only by the pharmacist so ordering.
* Only legend medicinal drugs may be prescribed by a pharmacist. Over-the-counter drugs are exempt from the requirements of this rule and shall be recommended as over-the-counter products.
* Pharmacy interns and technicians may not be involved in the ordering of the medicinal drugs permitted in this rule.

Prescription Refills
* No prescription may be filled or refilled in excess of one (1) year from the date of the original prescription was written.
* No prescription for a controlled substance listed in Schedule II may be refilled.
* No prescription for a controlled substance listed in Schedules III, IV, or V may be filled or refilled more than five (5) times within a period of six (6) months after the date on which the prescription was written.

Medicinal Drugs Which May Be Ordered by Pharmacists
A Pharmacist may order and dispense from the following formulary, within their professional judgment, subject to the stated conditions.
* Oral analgesics for mild to moderate pain. The pharmacist may order these drugs for minor pain and menstrual cramps for patients with no history of peptic

ulcer disease. The prescription shall be limited to a six (6) day supply for one treatment. If appropriate, the prescription shall be labeled to be taken with food or milk.
    - Magnesium salicylate/phenyltoloxamine citrate.
    - Acetylsalicylic acid (Zero order release, long acting tablets).
    - Choline salicylate and magnesium salicylate.
    - Naproxen sodium.
    - Naproxen.
    - Ibuprofen.
- Urinary analgesics. Phenazopyridine, not exceeding a two (2) day supply. The prescriptions shall be labeled about the tendency to discolor urine. If appropriate, the prescription shall be labeled to be taken after meals.
- Otic analgesics. Antipyrine 5.4%, benzocaine 1.4%, glycerin, if clinical signs or symptoms of tympanic membrane perforation do not exist. The product shall be labeled for use in the ear only.
- Anti-nausea preparations.
    - Meclizine up to 25 mg., except for a patient currently using a central nervous system (CNS) depressant. The prescription shall be labeled to advise the patient of drowsiness and to caution against concomitant use with alcohol or other depressants.
    - Scopolamine not exceeding 1.5 mg. per dermal patch. Patient shall be warned to seek appropriate medical attention if eye pain, redness or decreased vision develops.
- Antihistamines and decongestants. The following, including their salts, either as a single ingredient product or in combination, including nasal decongestants, may be ordered for a patient above 6 years of age.
    - Antihistamines. The pharmacist shall warn the patient that an antihistamine should not be used by patients with bronchial asthma or other lower

respiratory symptoms, glaucoma, cardiovascular disorders, hypertension, prostate conditions and urinary retention. An antihistamine shall be labeled to advise the patient of drowsiness and caution against the concomitant use with alcohol or other depressants.
- Diphenhydramine.
- Carbinoxamine.
- Pyrilamine.
- Dexchlorpheniramine.
- Brompheniramine.

  o Decongestants. The pharmacist shall not order an oral decongestant for use by a patient with coronary artery disease, angina, hyperthyroidism, diabetes, glaucoma, prostate conditions, hypertension, or a patient currently using a monoamine oxidase inhibitor.
- Phenylephrine.
- Azatadine.
- Topical antifungal/antibacterials. The pharmacist shall warn the patient that any of the products should not be used near deep or puncture wounds and contact with eyes or mucous membranes should be avoided. Iodochlorhydroxyquin preparations shall be labeled with staining potential.
  o Iodochlorhydroxyquin with 0.5% Hydrocortisone (not exceeding 20 grams).
  o Haloprogin 1%.
  o Clotrimazole topical cream and lotion.
  o Erythromycin topical.
- Topical anti-inflammatory. The pharmacist shall warn the patient that hydrocortisone should not be used on bacterial infections, viral infections, fungal infections, or by patients with impaired circulation. The prescription shall be labeled to advise the patient to avoid contact with eyes, mucous membranes or broken skin.

- Preparations containing hydrocortisone not exceeding 2.5%.
- Otic antifungal/antibacterial. Acetic acid 2% in aluminum acetate solution which shall be labeled for use in ears only.
- Keratolytics. Salicylic acid 16.7% and lactic acid 16.7% in flexible collodion, to be applied to warts, except for patients under two (2) years of age, and those with diabetes or impaired circulation. Prescriptions shall be labeled to avoid contact with normal skin, eyes and mucous membranes.
- Vitamins with fluoride. (This does not include vitamins with folic acid in excess of 0.9 mg.)
- Medicinal drug shampoos containing Lindane. The pharmacist shall:
  - Limit the order to the treatment of head lice only;
  - Order no more than four (4) ounces per person; and
  - Provide the patient with the appropriate instructions and precautions for use.
- Ophthalmics. Naphazoline 0.1% ophthalmic solution.
- Histamine H2 antagonists. The pharrmacist shall advise the patient to seek medical attention if symptom persist longer than 14 days while using the medication or if stools darken or contain blood.
  - Cimetidine.
  - Famotidine.
  - Ranitidine HC1.
- Acne products. Benzoyl Peroxide. The prescription shall be labeled to advise the patient to avoid use on the eye, eyelid, or mucous membranes.
- Topical Antiviral.
  - Acyclovir ointment may be ordered for the treatment of herpes simplex infections of the lips.
  - Penciclovir.

Fluoride Containing Products That May Be Ordered by Pharmacists
Oral medicinal drug products containing fluoride may be ordered by pharmacists for their patients who do not have fluoride supplement in their drinking water. Cannot change products (different manufacturer) once treatment has begun. Maximum of one year of treatment.

Standards of Practice - Continuous Quality Improvement Program
- "Continuous Quality Improvement Program" means a system of standards and procedures to identify and evaluate quality-related events and improve patient care.
- "Quality-Related Event" means the inappropriate dispensing or administration of a prescribed medication.
- Each pharmacy shall establish a Continuous Quality Improvement Program
- Quality-related events must be reviewed every 3 months

Registered Pharmacy Technician, to Pharmacist Ratio
- Pharmacist can only supervise one registered pharmacy technician unless otherwise permitted by the Florida Board of Pharmacy.
- Registered pharmacy technician must be under the direct personal supervision of a pharmacist

Registered Pharmacy Technician Responsibilities
- Registered pharmacy technicians may assist the pharmacist in performing the following tasks:
    - Retrieval of prescription files, patient files and profiles and other such records pertaining to the practice of pharmacy;
    - Data Entry;
    - Label preparation;

- The counting, weighing, measuring, pouring and compounding of prescription medication or stock legend drugs and controlled substances, including the filling of an automated medication system;
- Initiate communication to a prescribing practitioner or their medical staffs (or agents) regarding patient prescription refill authorization requests. For the purposes of this section "prescription refill" means the dispensing of medications pursuant to a prescriber's authorization provided on the original prescription;
- Initiate communication to confirm the patient's name, medication, strength, quantity, directions and date of last refill;
- Initiate communication to a prescribing practitioner or their medical staff (or agents) to obtain clarification on missing or illegible dates, prescriber name, brand/generic preference, quantity, DEA registration number or license numbers; and
- May accept authorization for a prescription renewal. For the purposes of this section, "prescription renewal" means the dispensing of medications pursuant to a practitioner's authorization to fill an existing prescription that has no refill remaining.

- Registered Pharmacy technicians shall not:
  - Receive new verbal prescriptions or any change in the medication, strength or directions;
  - Interpret a prescription or medication order for therapeutic acceptability and appropriateness;
  - Conduct a final verification of dosage and directions;
  - Engage in prospective drug review;
  - Provide patient counseling;
  - Monitor prescription usage; and

- o Override clinical alerts without first notifying the pharmacist.
- Nuclear pharmacy permits allow the registered pharmacy technician to receive diagnostic orders only. The pharmacist must receive therapy or blood product procedure orders.
- All registered pharmacy technicians shall identify themselves as registered pharmacy technicians by wearing a type of identification badge that is clearly visible which specifically identifies the employee by name and by status as a "registered pharmacy technician"; and
- All registered pharmacy technicians shall state their names and verbally identify themselves as registered pharmacy technicians in the context of telephone or other forms of communication.

Responsibilities of the Pharmacist

The delegation of any duties, tasks or functions to registered pharmacy interns and registered pharmacy technicians must be performed subject to a continuing review and ultimate supervision of the pharmacist who instigated the specific task, so that a continuity of supervised activity is present between one (1) pharmacist and one (1) registered pharmacy technician. In every pharmacy, the licensed pharmacist shall retain the professional and personal responsibility for any delegated act performed by registered pharmacy interns and registered pharmacy technicians in his employ and under his supervision.

Policies and Procedures

Must have policies and procedures in place regarding the number of registered pharmacy technicians and their utilization.

Negative Drug Formulary

The negative drug formulary is composed of medicinal drugs which have been specifically determined by the Board of Pharmacy and the Board of Medicine to demonstrate clinically significant biological or therapeutic inequivalence and which, if substituted, could produce adverse clinical effects, or could otherwise pose a threat to the health and safety of patients receiving such prescription medications. Except where certain dosage forms are included on the negative drug formulary as a class, all medicinal drugs are listed by their official United States Pharmacopoeia Non-Proprietary (generic) name. The generic name of a drug shall be applicable to and include all brand-name equivalents of such drug for which a prescriber may write a prescription. Substitution by a dispensing pharmacist on a prescription written for any brand name equivalent of a generic named drug product listed on the negative formulary or for a drug within the class of certain dosage forms as listed, is strictly prohibited. In cases where the prescription is written for a drug listed on the negative drug formulary but a brand name equivalent is not specified by the prescriber, the drug dispensed must be one obtained from a manufacturer or distributor holding an approved new drug application or abbreviated new drug application issued by the Food and Drug Administration, United States Department of Health and Welfare permitting that manufacturer or distributor to market those medicinal drugs or when the former is non-applicable, those manufacturers or distributors supplying such medicinal drugs must show compliance with other applicable Federal Food and Drug Administration marketing requirements. The following are included on the negative drug formulary:

- Digitoxin
- Conjugated Estrogen
- Dicumarol
- Chlorpromazine (Solid Oral Dosage Forms)
- Theophylline (Controlled Release)
- Pancrelipase (Oral Dosage Forms)

Identification of Manufacturer
Each formulary of generic and brand name drug products established by each community pharmacy shall include the

name of the manufacturer of the generic drug listed in said formulary.

Positive Drug Formulary
A positive formulary of generic and brand name drug products is required of each community pharmacy. Those medicinal drugs on the positive formulary shall be obtained from manufacturers or distributors holding an approved new drug application or abbreviated new drug application issued by the Food and Drug Administration, U.S. Department of Health, Education and Welfare permitting that manufacturer or distributor to market those medicinal drugs or when the former is non-applicable, those manufacturers or distributors supplying those medicinal drugs must show compliance with other applicable Federal Food and Drug Administration marketing requirements.

Duty of Pharmacist to Inform Regarding Drug Substitution
Prior to the delivery of the prescription, a pharmacist must inform the person presenting a prescription of any substitution of a generic drug product for a brand name drug product, of any retail price difference between the two, and of the person's right to refuse the substitution. This information must be communicated at a meaningful time such as to allow the person to make an informed choice as to whether to exercise the option to refuse substitution without undue inconvenience to the presenter of the prescription or to the consumer of the drug.

Possession and Disposition of Sample Medicinal Drugs
Pharmacies may not be in possession of sample medicinal drugs except:
- Pharmacies may possess the sample medicinal drugs that are listed within Rule 64B16-27.220, F.A.C., Medicinal Drugs That May be Ordered by Pharmacists.

- Institutional pharmacies may possess sample medicinal drugs upon the written request of the prescribing practitioner.
- Those community pharmacies that are pharmacies of health care entities, as defined by Sections 499.003(3), may possess sample medicinal drugs upon the written request of the prescribing practitioner.

Definition of Compounding

"Compounding" is the professional act by a pharmacist or other practitioner authorized by law, employing the science or art of any branch of the profession of pharmacy, incorporating ingredients to create a finished product for dispensing to a patient or for administration by a practitioner or the practitioner's agent; and shall specifically include the professional act of preparing a unique finished product containing any ingredient or device defined by Sections 465.003(7) and (8), F.S. The term also includes the preparation of nuclear pharmaceuticals and diagnostic kits incident to use of such nuclear pharmaceuticals. The term "commercially available products," as used in this section, means any medicinal product as defined by Sections 465.003(7) and (8), F.S., that are legally distributed in the State of Florida by a drug manufacturer or wholesaler.

- Compounding includes:
    - The preparation of drugs or devices in anticipation of prescriptions based on routine, regularly observed prescribing patterns.
    - The preparation pursuant to a prescription of drugs or devices which are not commercially available.
    - The preparation of commercially available products from bulk when the prescribing practitioner has prescribed the compounded product on a per prescription basis and the patient has been made aware that the compounded product will be prepared by the

pharmacist. The reconstitution of commercially available products pursuant to the manufacturer's guidelines is permissible without notice to the practitioner.
- The preparation of drugs or devices for sale or transfer to pharmacies, practitioners, or entities for purposes of dispensing or distribution is not compounding and is not within the practice of the profession of pharmacy. Except that the supply of patient specific compounded prescriptions to another pharmacy under the provisions of Section 465.0265, F.S., and Rule 64B16-28.450, F.A.C., is authorized.
- Office use compounding, "Office use" means the provision and administration of a compounded drug to a patient by a practitioner in the practitioner's office or by the practitioner in a health care facility or treatment setting, including a hospital, ambulatory surgical center, or pharmacy. A pharmacist may dispense and deliver a quantity of a compounded drug to a practitioner for office use by the practitioner in accordance with this section provided:
    o The quantity of compounded drug does not exceed the amount a practitioner anticipates may be used in the practitioner's office before the expiration date of the drug;
    o The quantity of compounded drug is reasonable considering the intended use of the compounded drug and the nature of the practitioner's practice;
    o The quantity of compounded drug for any practitioner and all practitioners as a whole, is not greater than an amount the pharmacy is capable of compounding in compliance with pharmaceutical standards for identity, strength, quality, and purity of the compounded drug that are consistent with United States Pharmacopoeia guidelines and accreditation practices.

Standards of Practice for Compounding Sterile Preparations (CSPs)

- The purpose of this section is to assure positive patient outcomes through the provision of standards for 1) pharmaceutical care; 2) the preparation, labeling, and distribution of sterile pharmaceuticals by pharmacies, pursuant to or in anticipation of a prescription drug order, and 3) product quality and characteristics. These standards are intended to apply to all sterile pharmaceuticals, notwithstanding the location of the patient (e.g., home, hospital, nursing home, hospice, doctor's office).
- Compounded sterile preparations include, but are not limited, to the following:
    - Total Parenteral Nutrition (TPN) solutions;
    - Parenteral analgesic drugs;
    - Parenteral antibiotics;
    - Parenteral antineoplastic agents;
    - Parenteral electrolytes;
    - Parenteral vitamins;
    - Irrigating fluids;
    - Ophthalmic preparations; and
    - Aqueous inhalant solutions for respiratory treatments.
- Sterile preparations shall not include commercially manufactured products that do not require compounding prior to dispensing.
- Policy & Procedure Manual. A policy and procedure manual shall be prepared and maintained for the compounding, dispensing, and delivery of sterile preparation prescriptions. The policy and procedure manual shall be available for inspection by the Department and include at a minimum:
    - Use of single dose and multiple dose containers not to exceed United States Pharmacopeia 797 guidelines.

- Verification of compounding accuracy and sterility.
- Personnel training and evaluation in aseptic manipulation skills.
- Environmental quality and control:
  - Air particle monitoring for hoods (or Barrier Isolator), clean room and buffer area (or anteroom) when applicable;
  - Unidirectional airflow (pressure differential monitoring);
  - Cleaning and disinfecting the sterile compounding areas;
  - Personnel cleansing and garbing;
  - Environmental monitoring (air and surfaces).
- Personnel monitoring and validation.
- Finished product checks and tests.
- Method to identify and verify ingredients used in compounding.
- Labeling requirements for bulk compounded products:
  - Contents;
  - Beyond-Use-Date; and
  - Storage requirements.
- Packing, storage, and transportation conditions.

- The pharmacy shall have a designated area with entry restricted to designated personnel for preparing parenteral products. This area shall have a specified ante area and buffer area; in high risk compounding, this shall be separate rooms. This area shall be structurally isolated from other areas with restricted entry or access, and must be designed to avoid unnecessary traffic and interference with unidirectional airflow. It shall be used only for the preparation of these sterile preparations. It shall be of sufficient size to accommodate a laminar airflow hood and to provide for the proper storage of drugs and supplies under appropriate conditions of temperature, light, moisture, sanitation, ventilation, and security.

- The pharmacy compounding parenteral and sterile preparation shall have the following:
    - Appropriate environmental control devices capable of maintaining at least class 100 conditions in the work place where critical objects are exposed and critical activities are performed; furthermore, these devices must be capable of maintaining class 100 conditions during normal activity. Examples of appropriate devices include laminar airflow hoods and zonal laminar flow of high efficiency particulate air (HEPA) filtered air;
    - Appropriate disposal containers for used needles, syringes, and if applicable, for antineoplastic waste from the preparation of chemotherapy agents;
    - Appropriate environmental control including approved biohazard cabinetry when antineoplastic drug products are prepared;
    - Appropriate temperature and transport containers;
    - Infusion devices and equipment, if appropriate.
- The pharmacy shall maintain and use supplies adequate to preserve an environment suitable for the aseptic preparation of sterile preparations, such as:
    - Gloves, masks, shoe covers, head and facial hair covers, and non-shedding gowns;
    - Needles and syringes of various standard sizes;
    - Disinfectant cleaning agents;
    - Clean towels;
    - Hand washing materials with bactericidal properties;
    - Vacuum containers and various transfer sets;
    - "Spill kits" for antineoplastic agent spills.

- The pharmacy should have current reference material in hard copy or readily available on line:
  - USP Pharmacist Pharmacopeia (optional) or Handbook of Injectable Drugs by American Society of Hospital Pharmacists; or other nationally recognized standard reference; and
  - "Practice Guidelines for Personnel Dealing with Cytotoxic Drugs," or other nationally recognized standard cytotoxic reference if applicable.
- Barrier isolator is exempt from all physical requirements subject to manufacturer guidelines for proper placement.

Antineoplastic Drugs. The following requirements are necessary for those pharmacies that prepare antineoplastic drugs to ensure the protection of the personnel involved:

- All antineoplastic drugs shall be compounded in a vertical flow, Class II, biological safety cabinet placed in negative pressure room unless using barrier isolators. Other preparations shall not be compounded in this cabinet.
- Protective apparel shall be worn by personnel compounding antineoplastic drugs. This shall include at least gloves and gowns with tight cuffs.
- Appropriate safety and containment techniques for compounding antineoplastic drugs shall be used in conjunction with the aseptic techniques required for preparing sterile products.
- Disposal of antineoplastic waste shall comply with all applicable local, state, and federal requirements.
- Written procedures for handling both major and minor spills of antineoplastic agents shall be developed and shall be included in the policy and procedure manual.
- Prepared doses of antineoplastic drugs shall be dispensed, labeled with proper precautions inside and outside, and shipped in a manner to minimize the risk of accidental rupture of the primary container.

Quality Assurance:

- There shall be a documented, ongoing quality assurance control program that monitors personnel performance, equipment, and preparations. Appropriate samples of finished preparations shall be examined to assure that the pharmacy is capable of consistently preparing sterile preparations meeting specifications:
    - All clean rooms and laminar flow hoods shall be certified by an independent contractor or National Sanitation Foundation Standard 49, for operational efficiency at least semiannually for high risk CSPs and annually for low and medium risk CSPs or any time the hood is relocated or the structure is altered and records shall be maintained for two years.
    - There shall be written procedures developed requiring sampling if microbial contamination is suspected for batches greater than 25 units.
    - High risk greater than 25 units have antimicrobial testing prior to dispensing.
    - There shall be referenced written justification of the chosen beyond-use-dates for compounded products.
    - There shall be documentation of quality assurance audits at regular planned intervals, including infection control and sterile technique audits.
- Compounding personnel shall be adequately skilled, educated, instructed, and trained to correctly perform and document the following activities in their sterile compounding duties:
    - Demonstrate by observation or test a functional understanding of USP Chapter 797 and definitions, to include Risk Category assessment;
    - Understand the characteristics of touch contamination and airborne microbial contaminants;
    - Perform antiseptic hand cleaning and disinfections of non-sterile compounding surfaces;

- Select and appropriately don protective garb;
- Demonstrate aseptic techniques and requirements while handling medications;
- Maintain and achieve sterility of CSPs in ISO Class 5 (Class 100) primary engineering devices and protect personnel and compounding environments from contamination by antineoplastic and chemotoxic or other hazardous drugs or substances;
- Manipulate sterile products aseptically, sterilize high-risk level CSPs (where applicable) and quality inspect CSPs;
- Identify, weigh and measure ingredients;
- Prepare product labeling requirements and "beyond use" requirements of product expiration;
- Prepare equipment and barrier requirement work requirements to maintain sterility;
- Prepare end point testing and demonstrated competencies for relevant risk levels;
- Prepare media fills to test aseptic technique.

Radiopharmaceuticals as Compounded Sterile Products
- Upon release of a Positron Emission Tomography (PET) radiopharmaceutical as a finished drug product from a PET production facility, the further manipulation, handling, or use of the product will be considered compounding and will be subject to the rules of this section.
- Radiopharmaceuticals compounded from sterile components in closed, sterile containers and with a volume of 100 ml or less for single dose injection or not more than 30 ml taken from a multiple dose container, shall be designated as, and conform to, the standards for low risk compounding.
- Radiopharmaceuticals shall be compounded using appropriately shielded vials and syringes in a properly functioning ISO Class 5 PEC (Primary Engineering Control), located in an ISO Class 8 or better buffer area

173

- environment in compliance with special handling, shielding, air flow requirements, and radiation safety programs to maintain radiation exposure as low as reasonably achievable.
- Radiopharmaceuticals designed for multi use, compounded with Tc-99m, exposed to an ISO Class 5 environment by components with no direct contact contamination, may be used up until the time indicated by manufacturers recommendations.
- Technetium 99/Molybdnenum 99 generator systems shall be stored and eluted in an ISO Class 8 or cleaner environment to permit special handling, shielding, and airflow requirements.
- Manipulation of blood or blood derived products (e.g. radiolabeling white blood cells) shall be conducted in an area that is clearly separated from routine material handling areas and equipment, and shall be controlled by specific standard operating procedures to avoid cross contamination of products. The buffer area for manipulation of blood or blood derived products shall be maintained as an ISO 7 environment and direct manipulations shall occur in an ISO 5 PEC suitable for these products (e.g. biological safety cabinet).

Requirement for Patient Records

The pharmacist shall ensure that a reasonable effort is made to obtain, record and maintain for at least 2 years the following information:
- Full name of the patient for whom the drug is intended
- Address and telephone number of the patient
- Patient's age or date of birth
- Patient's gender
- A list of all new and refill prescriptions obtained by the patient at the pharmacy maintaining the patient record during the two years immediately preceding the most recent entry showing the name of the drug or device, prescription number, name and strength of the drug, the

quantity and date received, and the name of the prescriber; and
- Pharmacist comments relevant to the individual's drug therapy, including any other information peculiar to the specific patient or drug.

Prospective Drug Use Review
Must be done by a pharmacist with each new and refill prescription:
- Over-utilization or under-utilization
- Therapeutic duplication
- Drug-disease contraindications
- Drug-drug interactions
- Incorrect drug dosage or duration of drug treatment
- Drug-allergy interactions
- Clinical abuse/misuse

Patient Counseling
- A verbal and printed offer to counsel must be done with each new or refill prescription
- Pharmacy intern may counsel if acting under the direct and immediate personal supervision of a licensed pharmacist
- If prescription mailed, then the offer must be in writing and include a toll-free telephone access to the pharmacist
- Counseling not required for inpatients of a hospital or institution where other licensed health care practitioners are authorized to administer the drug(s)
- Do not have to counsel if patient refuses

Standards of Practice - Drug Therapy Management
- "Prescriber Care Plan" means an individualized assessment of a patient and orders for specific drugs, laboratory tests, and other pharmaceutical services intended to be dispensed or executed by a pharmacist. The Prescriber Care Plan shall be written by a physician

licensed pursuant to Chapter 458, 459, 461, or 466, F.S., or similar statutory provision in another jurisdiction, and may be transmitted by any means of communication. The Prescriber Care Plan shall specify the conditions under which a pharmacist shall order laboratory tests, interpret laboratory values ordered for a patient, execute drug therapy orders for a patient, and notify the physician.

- "Drug Therapy Management" means any act or service by a pharmacist in compliance with orders in a Prescriber Care Plan.
- A pharmacist may provide Drug Therapy Management services for a patient, incidental to the dispensing of medicinal drugs or as a part of consulting concerning therapeutic values of medicinal drugs or as part of managing and monitoring the patient's drug therapy. A pharmacist who provides Drug Therapy Management services for a patient shall comply with orders in a Prescriber Care Plan, insofar as they specify:
    - Drug therapy to be initially dispensed to the patient by the pharmacist; or
    - Laboratory values or tests to be ordered, monitored and interpreted by the pharmacist; or
    - The conditions under which the duly licensed practitioner authorizes the execution of subsequent orders concerning the drug therapy for the patient; or
    - The conditions under which the pharmacist shall contact or notify the physician.
- A pharmacist who provides Drug Therapy Management services shall do so only under the auspices of a pharmacy permit that provides the following:
    - A transferable patient care record that includes:
        - A Prescriber Care Plan that includes a section noted as "orders" from a duly licensed physician for each patient for whom a pharmacist provides Drug Therapy Management services;

- - Progress notes; and
  - A pharmaceutical care area that is private, distinct, and partitioned from any area in which activities other than patient care activities occur, and in which the pharmacist and patient may sit down during the provision of Drug Therapy Management services; and
  - A continuous quality improvement program that includes standards and procedures to identify, evaluate, and constantly improve Drug Therapy Management services provided by a pharmacist.

Standards of Practice for the Dispensing of Controlled Substances for Treatment of Pain

- Cannot fill a prescription that is not issued for a legitimate medical purpose
- If the pharmacist believes it is not for a legitimate medical purpose they need to
  - Photocopy the patient's picture identification
  - Verify the prescription with the prescriber. A pharmacist who believes a prescription for a controlled substance medication to be valid, but who has not been able to verify it with the prescriber, may determine not to supply the full quantity and may dispense a partial supply, not to exceed a 72 hour supply. After verification by the prescriber, the pharmacist may dispense the balance of the prescription within a 72 hour time period following the initial partial filling.
- Every pharmacy permit holder shall maintain a computerized record of controlled substance prescriptions dispensed. A hard copy printout summary of such record, covering the previous 60 day period, shall be made available within 72 hours following a request for it by any law enforcement personnel.

Prescription Area Accessible to Inspection
- Can inspect anywhere prescriptions are compounded, filled, processed, accepted, dispensed, or stored
- Also can inspect invoices, shipping tickets, or any other document pertaining to the transfer of drugs or drug preparations, from or to all pharmacies
- There shall be a minimum of one (1) inspection per year except as otherwise provided herein or directed by the Board.
    - A pharmacy shall be inspected twice during the first year of operation.
    - A pharmacy which has had passing inspections for the most current three years, and no discipline during the most current three years shall be inspected every two years.
    - A pharmacy which fails to obtain a passing inspection or which is disciplined during the two year inspection cycle will be inspected annually until it achieves passing inspections for the most current three years, and no discipline during the most current three years as set forth in this subsection.

Sink and Running Water, Sufficient Space, Refrigeration, Sanitation, Equipment

There shall be provided for the prescription department of each pharmacy:
- Sink with running water
- Refrigerator
- Adequate sanitation to insure the prescription department is operating under clean, sanitary, uncrowded, and healthy conditions
- Electronic or hardcopy library of
    - A current pharmacy reference compendium such as the United States Pharmacopoeia/National Formulary, the U.S. Dispensatory, USP DI, (United States Pharmacopoeial Drug Information), the

Remington Practice of Pharmacy, Facts and Comparisons or an equivalent thereof sufficient in scope to meet the professional practice needs of that pharmacy
- Current copy of the laws and rules governing the practice of pharmacy in the State of Florida.

Patient Consultation Area

A community pharmacy shall provide a private consultation area so all patients of the pharmacy will be able to obtain counseling without being overheard by others in the prescription dispensing area of the pharmacy. The consultation area must be accessible by the patient from the outside of the prescription dispensing area of the pharmacy without having to traverse a stockroom or the prescription dispensing area. In determining whether the area is suitable, consideration shall be given to the proximity of the counseling area to the check-out or cash register area, the volume of pedestrian traffic in and around the consultation area, and the presence of walls or other barriers between the counseling area and the prescription dispensing area of the pharmacy. The consultation area may consist of designated private counter space. The area shall be designated with a sign bearing "Patient Consultation Area", or words that are substantially similar.

All Permits – Labels and Labeling of Medicinal Drugs

- Definitions.
    - "Controlled substance" means any substance named or described in Schedules II-V.
    - "Customized medication package" means a package that:
        - Is prepared by a pharmacist for a specific patient.
        - Is a series of containers.
        - Contains two (2) or more solid oral dosage forms.

- "Labeling" means a label or other written, printed, or graphic material upon an agent or product or any of its containers, wrappers, drug carts, or compartments thereof, as well as a medication administration record (MAR) if a medication administration record is an integral part of the unit dose system.
  - "Radiopharmaceutical" means any substance defined as a drug which exhibits spontaneous disintegration of unstable nuclei with the emission of nuclear particles or photons and includes any of those drugs intended to be made radioactive. This includes nonradioactive reagent kits and nuclide generators which are intended to be used in the preparation of any such substance, but does not include drugs which are carbon-containing compounds or potassium-containing compounds or potassium-containing salts which contain trace quantities of naturally occurring radionuclides.
  - "Serial number" means a prescription number or other unique number by which a particular prescription or drug package can be identified.
- The label affixed to each container dispensed to a patient shall include:
  - Name and address of the pharmacy.
  - Date of dispensing.
  - Serial number.
  - Name of the patient or, if the patient is an animal, the name of the owner and the species of animal.
  - Name of the prescriber.
  - Name of the drug dispensed (except where the prescribing practitioner specifically requests that the name is to be withheld).
  - Directions for use.
  - Expiration date.

- If the medicinal drug is a controlled substance, a warning that it is a crime to transfer the drug to another person.
- The label on the immediate container of a repackaged product or a multiple unit prepackaged drug product shall include
    - Brand or generic name.
    - Strength.
    - Dosage form.
    - Name of the manufacturer.
    - Expiration date.
    - Lot number:
        - Manufacturer's lot number, or
        - Number assigned by the dispenser or repackager which references the manufacturer's lot number.
- A medicinal drug dispensed in a unit dose system by a pharmacist shall be accompanied by labeling. The requirement will be satisfied if, to the extent not included on the label, the unit dose system indicates clearly the name of the resident or patient, the prescription number or other means utilized for readily retrieving the medication order, the directions for use, and the prescriber's name.
- A unit dose system shall provide a method for the separation and identification of drugs for the individual resident or patient.
- A customized patient medication package may be utilized if:
    - The consent of the patient or the patient's agent has been secured, and
    - The label includes:
        - Name, address and telephone number of the pharmacy.
        - Serial number for the customized medication package and a separate serial number for each medicinal drug dispensed.

- Date of preparation of the customized patient medication package.
- Patient's name.
- Name of each prescriber.
- Directions for use and any cautionary statements required for each medicinal drug.
- Storage instructions.
- Name, strength, quantity and physical description of each drug product.
- A beyond use date that is not more than 60 days from the date of preparation of the customized patient medication package but shall not be later than any appropriate beyond use date for any medicinal drug included in the customized patient medication package.
  - The customized patient medication package can be separated into individual medicinal drug containers, then each container shall identify the medicinal drug product contained.
- The label affixed to the immediate outer container shield of a radiopharmaceutical shall include:
  - Name and address of the pharmacy.
  - Name of the prescriber.
  - Date of the original dispensing.
  - The standard radiation symbol.
  - The words "Caution Radioactive Material."
  - Name of the procedure.
  - Prescription order number.
  - Radionuclide and chemical form.
  - Amount of radioactivity and the calibration date and time.
  - Expiration date and time.
  - If a liquid, the volume.
  - If a solid, the number of items or weight
  - If a gas, the number of ampules or vials.

- o Molybdenum 99 content to the United States Pharmacopeia (UPS) limits.
  - o Name of the patient or the words "Physician's Use Only."
- The label affixed to the immediate inner container of a radiopharmaceutical to be distributed shall include:
  - o The standard radiation symbol.
  - o The words "Caution Radioactive Material."
  - o Radionuclide and chemical form.
  - o Name of the procedure.
  - o Prescription order number of the radiopharmaceutical.
  - o Name of the pharmacy.
- The labeling on a carton or package containing a medicinal drug or product dispensed from an Extended Scope Renal Dialysis (ESRD) pharmacy shall include:
  - o "Use as Directed" statement.
  - o The name and address of the person to whom the products will be delivered.
  - o Name of the prescriber.
  - o Name and address of the ESRD pharmacy location from which the products were shipped.
  - o Prescription number.
  - o Any special instructions regarding delivery dates or locations.
  - o Beyond use date or, if the medicinal drug or product is dispensed in an unopened sealed package, the manufacturer's expiration date.

Regulation of Daily Operating Hours
- Must keep a community pharmacy prescription department of the establishment open for a minimum of forty (40) hours per week. Maybe closed for major holidays.
- Must have a sign displaying hours shall be displayed either at the main entrance of the establishment or at or

near the place where prescriptions are dispensed in a prominent place that is in clear and unobstructed view.
- May receive approval for less than 40 hours but minimum of 20 hours per week required. Must have policy and procedure for transferring a prescription, or receiving an emergency dose during the time the pharmacy is open less than 40 hours.

Prescription Department; Padlock; Sign: "Prescription Department Closed."
- Prescription department is closed whenever there is not a pharmacist is not present and on duty. A sign will be displayed saying "Prescription Department Closed."
- Does not include when pharmacist is on a meal break, or assisting patients.
- At all times when the prescription department is closed, either because of the absence of a pharmacist or for any other reason, it shall be separated from the remainder of the establishment by partition or other means of enclosure, thereby preventing access to the prescription department by persons not licensed in Florida to practice the profession of pharmacy.
- The partition or other means of enclosure shall be securely locked or padlocked and only a pharmacist shall have the means to gain access to the prescription department.
- When the prescription department of any community pharmacy establishment is closed, no person other than a pharmacist shall enter, be permitted to enter or remain in the prescription department.

Outdated Pharmaceuticals
Must examine the stock of the prescription department at least every 4 months to remove expired drugs.

Unit Dose and Customized Patient Medication Package Returns by In-patients

No pharmacist shall place into the stock of any pharmacy permittee any part of any prescription, compounded or dispensed, which is returned by a patient except under the following conditions:

- In a closed drug delivery system in which unit dose or customized patient medication packages are dispensed to in-patients, the unused medication may be returned to the pharmacy for redispensing only if each unit dose or customized patient medication package is individually sealed and if each unit dose or the unit dose system, or the customized patient medication package container or the customized patient medication package unit of which it is clearly a part is labeled with the name of the drug, dosage strength, manufacturer's control number, and expiration date, if any.
- In the case of controlled substances, as it is allowed by Federal Law.
- A "unit dose system" to which this rule applies means a system wherein all individually sealed unit doses are physically connected as a unit. For purpose of this section, a product in an unopened, sealed, manufacture's container is deemed to be a unit dose package.
- A "customized patient medication package" to which this rule applies means a system wherein all USP approved multi-dose units are physically connected and are referred to as a container.
- A "closed drug delivery system" to which this rule applies is a system in which the actual control of the unit dose or customized patient medication package is maintained by the facility rather than by the individual patient.

Unclaimed Prescriptions

Unclaimed prescriptions maybe reused up to one year from date of filling or reaches the product's expiration date, whichever is first.

All Permits – Storage of Legend Drugs; Prepackaging

- All medicinal drugs or drug preparations shall be stored:
  - Within the confines of the prescription department of a community pharmacy
  - In a Class II Institutional pharmacy within the confines of the pharmacy provided, however, that those medicinal drugs established by the consultant pharmacist as supportive to treatment procedures such as medical drugs, surgical, obstetrical, diagnostic, etc., may be permitted to be stored in those areas where such treatment is conducted consistent with proper control procedures as provided by the policy and procedure manual of the pharmacy.
- All medicinal drugs or drug preparations within Class I Institutional permittees and Special ALF Permit shall:
  - Be administered from individual prescription containers to the individual patient; and
  - Be prohibited within the confines of Class I Institutional pharmacies unless obtained upon a proper prescription and properly labeled.
- Prepackaging of medication, whether a part of a unit dose system or a part of a multiple dose drug distribution system in an extended care facility or hospital holding a valid Class II Institutional pharmacy permit, must be done in accordance with procedures set up by the consultant pharmacist of record in the policy and procedure manual; and in the case of a pharmacy holding a valid community pharmacy permit must be done in accordance with procedures set up by the prescription department manager.
- Medicinal drugs and proprietary preparations as identified above that are stored in treatment areas must be accessible only to licensed staff (pharmacists, nurses, physicians, advanced registered nurse practitioners,

physician assistants, respiratory and physical therapist, radiology technicians and registered pharmacy technicians, etc.) in accordance with their license, practice act, or to other personnel specifically authorized by the institution.

Record Maintenance Systems for Community, Special-Limited Community, Special-Closed Systems, Special-Parenteral/Enteral, and Nuclear Permits

<u>Requirements for records maintained in a data processing system</u>

- Original prescriptions shall be reduced to a hard copy if not received in written form. All original prescriptions shall be retained for a period of not less than two years from date of last filling. A pharmacy may, in lieu of retaining the actual original prescriptions, use an electronic imaging recordkeeping system, provided such system is capable of capturing, storing, and reproducing the exact image of the prescription, including the reverse side of the prescription if necessary, and that such image be retained for a period of no less than two years from the date of last filling.
- Original prescriptions shall be maintained in a two or three file system.
- Requirements for back-up systems.
    - The pharmacy shall maintain a back-up copy of information stored in the data processing system using disk, tape or other electronic back-up system and update this back-up copy on a regular basis, at least weekly, to assure that data is not lost due to system failure.
- Maintain data for the preceding two years.
- Loss of Data. The prescription department manager shall report to the Board in writing any significant loss of information from the data processing system within 10 days of discovery of the loss.

Records of dispensing
- Each time a prescription drug order is filled or refilled, a record of such dispensing shall be entered into the data processing system.
- The data processing system shall have the capacity to produce a daily hard-copy printout of all original prescriptions dispensed and refilled. This hard copy printout shall contain the following information:
    - Unique identification number of the prescription;
    - Date of dispensing;
    - Patient name;
    - Prescribing practitioner's name;
    - Name and strength of the drug product actually dispensed, if generic name, the brand name or manufacturer of drug dispensed;
    - Quantity dispensed;
    - Initials or an identification code of the dispensing pharmacist; and
    - If not immediately retrievable via CRT display, the following shall also be included on the hard-copy printout:
        - Patient's address;
        - Prescribing practitioner's address;
        - Practitioner's DEA registration number, if the prescription drug order is for a controlled substance.
        - Quantity prescribed, if different from the quantity dispensed;
        - Date of issuance of the prescription drug order, if different from the date of dispensing; and
        - Total number of refills dispensed to date for that prescription drug order.
- The daily hard-copy printout shall be produced within 72 hours of the date on which the prescription drug orders were dispensed and shall be maintained in a separate file at the pharmacy. Records of controlled substances shall

- be readily retrievable from records of non-controlled substances.
- Each individual pharmacist who dispenses or refills a prescription drug order shall verify that the data indicated on the daily hard-copy printout is correct, by dating and signing such document in the same manner as signing a check or legal document (e.g., J.H. Smith, or John H. Smith) within seven days from the date of dispensing.
- In lieu of producing the printout described above, the pharmacy shall maintain a log book in which each individual pharmacist using the data processing system shall sign a statement each day, attesting to the fact that the information entered into the data processing system that day has been reviewed by him or her and is correct as entered. Must be kept for two years after the date of dispensing provided.
- The prescription department manager and the permit holder are responsible maintaining records.
- Failure to provide the records set out in this section, either on site or within 48 hours for whatever reason, constitutes failure to keep and maintain records.
- In the event that a pharmacy which uses a data processing system experiences system downtime, the following is applicable;
    - An auxiliary procedure shall ensure that refills are authorized by the original prescription drug order and that the maximum number of refills has not been exceeded or that authorization from the prescribing practitioner has been obtained prior to dispensing a refill; and
    - All of the appropriate data shall be retained for on-line data entry as soon as the system is available for use again.

<u>Compounding records.</u> A written record shall be maintained for each batch/sub-batch of a compounded product. This record shall include:
- Date of compounding.

- Control number for each batch/sub-batch of a compounded product. This may be the manufacture's lot number or new numbers assigned by the pharmacist. If the number is assigned by the pharmacist, the pharmacist shall also record the original manufacture's lot number and expiration dates. If the original numbers and expiration dates are not known, the pharmacy shall record the source and acquisition date of the component.
- A complete formula for the compounded product maintained in a readily retrievable form including methodology and necessary equipment.
- A signature or initials of the pharmacist or pharmacy technician performing the compounding.
- A signature or initials of the pharmacist responsible for supervising pharmacy technicians involved in the compounding process.
- The name(s) of the manufacturer(s) of the raw materials used.
- The quantity in units of finished products or grams of raw materials.
- The package size and number of units prepared.
- The name of the patient who received the particular compounded product.

Authorization of additional refills. Practitioner authorization for additional refills of a prescription drug order shall be noted as follows:
- On the daily hard-copy printout; or
- Via the CRT display.

Requirements for an Automated Pharmacy System in a Community Pharmacy

- Definitions. "Automated pharmacy system" means a mechanical system, located within or adjacent to the prescription department, that performs operations or activities, other than compounding or administration, relative to storage, packaging, dispensing, or distribution

of medication, and which collects, controls, and maintains all transaction information.
- General Requirements. A pharmacy may use an automated pharmacy system provided that:
  - The pharmacy develops and maintains a policy and procedure manual that includes:
    - The type or name of the system including a serial number or other identifying nomenclature.
    - A method to ensure security of the system to prevent unauthorized access. Such method may include the use of electronic passwords, biometric identification (optic scanning or fingerprint) or other coded identification.
    - A process of filling and stocking the system with drugs; an electronic or hard copy record of medication filled into the system including the product identification, lot number, and expiration date.
    - A method of identifying all the registered pharmacy interns or registered pharmacy technicians involved in the dispensing process.
    - Compliance with a Continuous Quality Improvement Program.
    - A method to ensure that patient confidentiality is maintained.
    - A process to enable the prescription department manager or designee to revoke, add, or change access at any time.
  - The system ensures that each prescription is dispensed in compliance with the definition of dispense and the practice of the profession of pharmacy.
  - The system shall maintain a readily retrievable electronic record to identify all pharmacists,

registered pharmacy technicians, or other personnel involved in the dispensing of a prescription.
- o The system shall provide the ability to comply with product recalls generated by the manufacturer, distributor, or pharmacy. The system shall have a process in place to isolate affected lot numbers including an intermix of drug product lot numbers.
- Additional Requirements for Patient Accessed Automated Pharmacy Systems. A pharmacy may use a patient accessed automated pharmacy system, provided that:
  - o Meets the requirements above.
  - o The stocking or restocking of a medicinal drug shall only be completed by a Florida pharmacist, except as provided in paragraph below.
  - o If the automated pharmacy system uses removable cartridges or container to store the drug, the stocking or restocking of the cartridges or containers may occur at a licensed repackaging facility and be sent to the provider pharmacy to be loaded by personnel designated by the pharmacist if:
    - A Florida pharmacist verifies the cartridge or container has been properly filled and labeled.
    - The individual cartridge or container is transported to the provider pharmacy in a secure, tamper-evident container.
    - The automated pharmacy system uses a bar code verification, electronic verification, weight verification, radio frequency identification (RFID) or similar process to ensure that the cartridge or container is accurately loaded into the automated pharmacy system.
    - The Florida pharmacist verifying the filling and labeling is responsible if the cartridge or container is stocked or restocked

- incorrectly by the personnel designated to load the cartridges or containers.
  - The automated pharmacy system must use at least two separate verifications, such as bar code verification, electronic verification, weight verification, radio frequency identification (RFID) or similar process to ensure that the proper medication is being dispensed from the automated system.
  - The medication shall bear a patient specific label that complies with Rule 64B16-28.108.
  - The record of transactions with the patient accessed automated pharmacy system shall be available to authorized agents of the Department of Health. The record of transactions shall include:
    - Name of the patient.
    - Name, strength, and dosage form of the drug product dispensed.
    - Quantity of drug dispensed.
    - Date and time of dispensing.
    - Name of provider pharmacy.
    - Prescription number.
    - Name of prescribing practitioner.
    - Identity of the pharmacist who approved the prescription or order.
    - Identity of the person to whom the drug was released.
- The Florida pharmacist responsible for filling, verifying, or loading the automated pharmacy system shall be responsible for her or his individual action.
- A prescription dispensed pursuant to the requirements of this rule shall be deemed to have been certified by the pharmacist.

Closing of a Pharmacy; Transfer of Prescription Files

- The term "prescription files" as used herein shall mean the drug dispensing records of a pharmacy which shall include all orders for drugs or medicinal supplies, inclusive of dispensing records for medicinal drugs, issued by a duly licensed practitioner, which serve to transfer possession of medicinal drugs from the pharmacy to the ultimate consumer.
- The term "closing of a pharmacy" as used herein shall mean the cessation or termination of professional and business activities within a pharmacy for which a permit has been issued.
- Prior to closure of a pharmacy the permittee shall notify the Board of Pharmacy in writing as to the effective date of closure, and shall:
    - Return the pharmacy permit to the Board of Pharmacy office or arrange with the local Bureau of Investigative Services of the Department to have the pharmacy permit returned to the Board of Pharmacy;
    - Advise the Board of Pharmacy which permittee is to receive the prescription files;
- On the date of closure of a pharmacy the former permittee shall:
    - Physically deliver the prescription files to a pharmacy operating within reasonable proximity of the pharmacy being closed and within the same locality. This delivery of prescription files may occur prior to the return of the pharmacy permit to the Board of Pharmacy office; and
    - Affix a prominent sign to the front entrance of the pharmacy advising the public of the new location of the former permittee's prescription files or otherwise provide a means by which to advise the public of the new location of their prescription files.

- After the closing of a pharmacy as defined herein, the custody of the prescription files of the pharmacy shall be transferred to the new permittee, unless the former permittee and the new permittee inform the Board in writing that custody of the prescription files have been or are to be transferred to a pharmacy other than the new permittee.
- A pharmacy receiving custody of prescription files from another pharmacy shall maintain the delivered prescriptions in separate files so as to prevent intermingling with the transferee pharmacy's prescription files.

Change of Ownership
- A pharmacy permit is not transferable. Upon the sale of an existing pharmacy, a new application must be filed. In those cases where the permit is held by a corporation, the transfer of all the stock of said corporation to another person or entity does not constitute a change of ownership, provided that the initial corporation holding the permit continues to exist.
- A change in ownership (and issuance of a new permit number) requires that new records be started and old records closed. The process for closing a pharmacy, including the transfer of prescription files and medicinal drugs must be followed for the old permit. If the old permit has controlled substances, the new permit must record an "opening inventory" for DEA purposes. Both the new permit and the old permit must keep appropriate records for two (2) years for the transfer of legend drugs and controlled substances.
- A change in the company or person who leases the building where the permit is housed or a change in the management company which contracts with the owner of the permit for the operation of the permit does not constitute a change in ownership.

Transfer of Medicinal Drugs; Change of Ownership; Closing of a Pharmacy

Ownership of medicinal drugs may be transferred to a new owner upon the change of ownership of a pharmacy or upon the closing of a pharmacy. The transferee entity acquiring ownership shall be authorized to prescribe, dispense or distribute such drugs. The transferor pharmacy shall provide the Florida Board of Pharmacy with the following information:

- The name, address, pharmacy permit number and D.E.A. registration number of the transferor pharmacy.
- The name, address, permit number, D.E.A. registration number (if available), and authorized business activity of the transferee entity.
- The date on which the transfer will occur.
- A complete inventory of all medicinal drugs as of the date of transfer. If the medicinal drug is listed in Schedule II, the transferor shall make an exact count or measure of the contents. If the medicinal drugs are listed in Schedule III, IV, or V, the transferor shall make an estimated count or measure of the contents, unless the container holds more than 1,000 tablets or capsules, in which case an exact count of the contents shall be made. This inventory shall serve as the final inventory of the permittee transferor and the transfer inventory of the transferee entity. The transferor and transferee shall each retain a copy of the inventory in their records and shall provide the Board of Pharmacy with a copy of such inventory. Transfer of any controlled substance in Schedule II shall require the use of order form, D.E.A. form number 222.
- Unless the permittee-transferor is informed by the Board of Pharmacy or the regional D.E.A. Administrator prior to the date on which the transfer was stated to occur, that the transfer may not occur, the permittee-transferor may proceed with the transfer.
- On the date of transfer of the medicinal drugs, all records required to be kept by the permittee-transferor of the transferred drugs which are controlled substances, shall

be transferred to the permittee-transferor. Responsibility for the accuracy of records prior to the date of transfer remains with the permittee-transferor, but responsibility for custody and maintenance shall be upon the permittee-transferee. It is the responsibility of the permittee-transferor to return all unused Schedule II order forms (D.E.A. form no. 222) to the regional D.E.A. office.

Destruction of Controlled Substances – Institutional Pharmacies

- Controlled substances that have been dispensed and not used by the patient shall not be returned to the pharmacy and shall be securely stored by the nursing home until destroyed.
- A document must be completed showing the name and quantity of the drug, strength and dosage form, patient's name, prescription number and name of the institution. This documentation, at the time of destruction, shall be witnessed and signed by the consultant pharmacist, director of nursing, and the administrator or his designee, which may include a licensed physician, pharmacists, mid-level practitioner, or nurse.

Destruction of Controlled Substances All Permittees (excluding Nursing Homes)

- Controlled substances that cannot be retained as usable shall be securely stored in the prescription department of the permittee pharmacy until destroyed.
- Permittees are required to complete a United States Drug Enforcement Administration (D.E.A.) Form 41. This form, at the time of destruction, shall be witnessed and signed by the prescription department manager or the consultant pharmacist of record and D.E.A. agent, or a Department inspector. This method of destruction does not require prior approval from D.E.A., but does require

that a copy of the completed and witnessed D.E.A. Form 41 be mailed to D.E.A. immediately after destruction.
- Another method of destruction shall be conducted by at least two persons who are either a licensed pharmacist, physician or nurse, or a sworn law enforcement officer or any combination thereof, to serve as the witnesses. A copy of the completed D.E.A. Form 41 and a letter providing the proposed date of destruction, the proposed method of destruction and the names and titles of the proposed witnesses must be received by D.E.A. at least two weeks prior to the proposed date of destruction which shall constitute a request for destruction. The drugs may not be destroyed until D.E.A. grants approval of the request for destruction. A copy of the completed and witnessed D.E.A. Form 41 shall be mailed to D.E.A. immediately after destruction.
- In lieu of destruction on the premises, controlled substances may also be shipped to reverse distributors for destruction in conformity with federal guidelines.

Centralized Prescription Filling, Delivering and Returning

- As used herein:
    - The term "originating pharmacy" means a pharmacy wherein the prescription which will be filled by the central fill pharmacy is initially presented; and
    - The term "central fill pharmacy" means a pharmacy which performs centralized prescription filling, delivering, and returning for one or more originating pharmacies.
- Pharmacies acting as the central fill pharmacy must be authorized to dispense medications under the provisions of Chapter 465, F.S.
- A community pharmacy which acts as the central fill pharmacy and which notifies the Board that its pharmacy

practice is limited only to such practice shall be exempt from the following rules:
- Rule 64B16-28.1035, F.A.C., Patient Consultation Area;
- The signage requirement of subsection 64B16-28.109(1), F.A.C.; and
- Rule 64B16-28.1081, F.A.C., Regulation of Daily Operating Hours.

- Delivery of medications. Delivery of medications must be made in a timely manner. The originating and central fill pharmacies shall each be identified on the prescription container.
  - Delivery by central fill pharmacy to ultimate consumer. A central fill pharmacy may deliver medications for an originating pharmacy to the ultimate consumer or the consumer's agent under the following conditions:
    - The pharmacies are under the same ownership or have a written contract specifying the services to be provided by each pharmacy, the responsibilities of each pharmacy, and the manner in which each pharmacy will comply with federal and state laws, rules and regulations.
    - The pharmacies shall have a pharmacist available 40 hours a week, either in person or via two-way communication technology, such as a telephone, to provide patient counseling.
    - The pharmacies shall include a toll-free number that allows the patient to reach a pharmacist for the purposes of patient counseling.
    - The pharmacies shall each be identified on the prescription container label. The originating pharmacy shall be identified with pharmacy name and address. The

central fill pharmacy may be identified by a code available at the originating pharmacy.
- The central fill pharmacy shall only deliver via carrier to the ultimate consumer or the consumer's agent those medications which could have been delivered via carrier by the originating pharmacy.
- The central fill pharmacy shall not deliver to the ultimate consumer or consumer's agent controlled substances.
  - The delivery of a filled prescription by a central fill pharmacy to the ultimate consumer or the consumer's agent pursuant to a contract with an originating pharmacy shall not be considered dispensing within the definition set forth in Section 465.003(6), F.S.
  - Each pharmacist that performs a specific function within the processing of the prescription shall be responsible for any errors or omissions committed by that pharmacist during the performance of that specific function.
- The supplying and receiving pharmacy shall each be identified on the prescription container label. The receiving pharmacy shall be identified with pharmacy name and address. The supplying pharmacy may be identified by a code available at the receiving pharmacy. Prescription and labeling requirements for pharmacies participating in central prescription filling, delivering and returning:
  - Prescriptions may be transmitted electronically from an originating pharmacy to a central fill pharmacy including via facsimile. The originating pharmacy transmitting the prescription information must:
    - Write the word "central fill" on the face of the original prescription and record the name, address, and DEA registration

number if a controlled substance of the originating pharmacy to which the prescription has been transmitted and the name of the originating pharmacy's pharmacist transmitting the prescription, and the date of transmittal;
- Ensure all the information required to be on a prescription pursuant to Sections 456.0392 and 893.04, F.S., is transmitted to the central fill pharmacy either on the face of the prescription or in the electronic transmission of information;
- Indicate in the information transmitted the number of refills already dispensed and the number of refills remaining;
- Maintain the original prescription for a period of two years from the date the prescription was last refilled.
- Keep a record of receipt of the filled prescription, including the date of receipt, the method of delivery (private, common or contract carrier) and the name of the originating pharmacy's employee accepting delivery.

o The central fill pharmacy receiving the transmitted prescription must:
- Keep a copy of the prescription if sent via facsimile, or an electronic record of all the information transmitted by the originating pharmacy, including the name, address, and DEA registration number, if a controlled substance, of the originating pharmacy transmitting the prescription;
- Keep a record of the date of receipt of the transmitted prescription, the name of the licensed pharmacist filling the

- prescription, and dates of filling or refilling of the prescription;
- Keep a record of the date the filled prescription was delivered to the originating pharmacy and the method of delivery (private, common or contract carrier).
- A central fill pharmacy's pharmacist filling a written or emergency oral prescription for a controlled substance listed in Schedule II shall affix to the package a label showing the date of filling, the receiving pharmacy's name and address, a unique identifier (i.e. the supplying pharmacy's DEA registration number) indicating the prescription was filled at the central fill pharmacy, the serial number of the prescription, the name of the patient, the name of the prescribing practitioner, and directions for use and cautionary statements, if any, contained in such prescription or required by law.

Pharmacy Common Database

- A pharmacy licensed under this chapter may perform prescription drug processing for other pharmacies, provided that all pharmacies are under common ownership, utilize a common database, and are properly licensed, permitted or registered in this state or another state. Nothing in this subsection shall prohibit a pharmacist employee of said pharmacies who is licensed in Florida or in another state from remotely accessing the pharmacy's electronic database from outside the pharmacy in order to process prescriptions, provided the pharmacy establishes controls to protect the privacy and security of confidential records.

- Prescription drug processing shall include the following:
    - Receiving, interpreting, or clarifying a prescription;
    - Entering prescription data into the pharmacy's record;
    - Verifying or validating a prescription;
    - Performing prospective drug review as defined by the Board;
    - Obtaining refill and substitution authorizations;
    - Interpreting or acting on clinical data;
    - Performing therapeutic interventions;
    - Providing drug information concerning a patient's prescription; and
    - Providing patient counseling.
- Each pharmacist that performs a specific function within the prescription drug processing process via use of a common database shall be responsible for any errors or omissions committed by that pharmacist during the performance of that specific function.
- Each pharmacy performing prescription drug processing pursuant to this section must maintain a policy and procedure manual, which shall be made available to the Board or its agent upon request. The policy and procedures manual shall include the following information:
    - A description for how each pharmacy will comply with federal and state laws, rules and regulations;
    - The procedure for maintaining appropriate records to identify the pharmacies and pharmacists responsible for the prescription drug processing and dispensing of the prescription;
    - The policy and procedure for providing adequate security to protect the confidentiality and integrity of patient information; and
    - The procedure to be used by the pharmacy in implementing and operating a quality assurance program designed to objectively and

- systematically monitor, evaluate, and improve the quality and appropriateness of patient care.
- The prescription drug processing of a prescription by one pharmacy for another pursuant to this section shall not be construed as the transferring of a prescription as set forth in Section 465.026, F.S.
- In addition to all record requirements of Rule 64B16-28.140, F.A.C., all pharmacies participating in prescription drug processing, shall maintain appropriate records which identify, by prescription, the name(s), initials, or identification code(s) of each pharmacist or registered pharmacy technician who performs a processing function for a prescription. Such records shall be maintained:
  - Separately by each pharmacy and pharmacist; or
  - In a common electronic file, as long as the records are maintained in such a manner that the data processing system can produce a printout which lists the functions performed by each pharmacy, pharmacist, registered pharmacy intern and registered pharmacy technician.

Institutional Permit – Consultant Pharmacist of Record

Each facility holding a Class I, a Class II, or a Modified Class II Institutional permit shall designate a consultant pharmacist of record to ensure compliance with the laws and rules governing the permit. The Board office shall be notified in writing within 10 days of any change in the consultant pharmacist of record. The consultant pharmacist of record for a Class I, Modified Class II, or a Special ALF permit shall conduct Drug Regimen Reviews as required by Federal or State law, inspect the facility and prepare a written report to be filed at the permitted facility at least monthly. In addition, the consultant pharmacist of record must monitor monthly the facility system for providing medication administration records and physician order sheets to ensure that the most current record of medications is available for the monthly drug regimen review. The consultant pharmacist of record may utilize additional consultant pharmacists to assist in this review and or in the monthly facility inspection.

Class I Institutional Permit and Class II Institutional Permit – Labels and Labeling of Medicinal Drugs for Inpatients of a Nursing Home

- The label affixed to a container used in conventional dispensing to a Class I Institutional permit or a Class II Institutional permit which, within the scope of its practice, services only the inpatients of a nursing home, shall contain at least the following information:
    - The name of and address of the pharmacy;
    - The name of the prescriber;
    - The name of the patient;
    - The date of the original filling or the refill date;
    - The prescription number or other prescription identification adequate to readily identify the prescription;
    - The directions for use;
    - The name of the medicinal drug dispensed (except where the health care practitioner prescribing the drug specifically denotes that the name is to be withheld).
    - The quantity of the drug in the container.
- The label affixed to a container used in dispensing controlled substances listed, in regard to conventional dispensing shall contain at least the following information:
    - All of the above information is required;
    - The number of the prescription as recorded in the prescription files of the pharmacy in which it is filled; and
    - A clear, concise warning that it is a crime to transfer the controlled substance to any person other than the patient for whom prescribed.

Transmission of Starter Dose Prescriptions for Patients in Class I Institutional or Modified II B Facilities

- Definitions.
    - "Vendor pharmacy" means a community pharmacy or special closed system pharmacy which has a contract to dispense a medicinal drug to a patient in a facility holding a Class I Institutional Permit or Modified II B Permit.
    - "Starter dose pharmacy" means a pharmacy that dispenses a medicinal drug pursuant to a starter dose prescription to a patient in a facility served by the vendor pharmacy.
    - "Starter dose prescription" means a prescription transmitted by a vendor pharmacy to a starter dose pharmacy for the purpose of initiating drug therapy for a patient in a facility served by the vendor pharmacy.
- A vendor pharmacy may transmit a starter dose prescription to a starter dose pharmacy if the vendor pharmacy:
    - Has written authorization from the facility to utilize a starter dose pharmacy.
    - Has a written contract with the starter dose pharmacy.
    - Has written authorization from a prescribing practitioner to act as the practitioner's agent for the purpose of transmitting a starter dose prescription.
    - Possess a valid prescription from the prescribing practitioner prior to transmitting the starter dose prescription.
    - Maintains a record of each starter dose prescription.
    - Maintains a policy and procedure manual that references starter dose prescriptions.

- A starter dose pharmacy may dispense a medicinal drug pursuant to a starter dose prescription for a patient in a facility that holds a Class I Institutional Permit or Modified II B Permit if the starter dose pharmacy:
    o Has a written contract with the vendor pharmacy.
    o Maintains a record of each starter dose prescription.
    o Maintains a policy and procedure manual that references starter dose prescriptions.
- The contract between a vendor pharmacy and a prescribing practitioner shall:
    o Be in writing.
    o Identify each facility served by the vendor pharmacy for which the authorization is valid.
    o Authorize the vendor pharmacy to transmit, as an agent of the practitioner, a starter dose prescription to a starter dose pharmacy.
    o Be on file at the vendor pharmacy, at the facility served by the vendor pharmacy, and with the prescribing practitioner.
    o Be available for inspection by agents of the Department of Health or the Board of Pharmacy.
- The contract between the vendor pharmacy and the starter dose pharmacy shall:
    o Be in writing.
    o Identify each facility served by the vendor pharmacy.
    o Assign the responsibility for prospective drug use review required by Rule 64B16-27.810, F.A.C., to the vendor pharmacy.
    o Assign the responsibility for patient counseling required by Rule 64B16-27.820, F.A.C., to the vendor pharmacy.
    o Be referenced in the Policy and Procedure Manual of the vendor pharmacy and of the starter dose pharmacy.

- - Be updated as necessary to identify facilities or practitioners.
  - Be on file at the vendor pharmacy, at the starter dose pharmacy, and at the facility.
  - Be available for inspection by authorized agents of the Department of Health and the Board of Pharmacy.
- A record of each starter dose prescription shall be:
  - Readily retrievable.
  - Maintained for two years.

Institutional Class II Dispensing

- Pharmaceutical preparations which are administered to patients of a hospital by the personnel of such institution shall only be taken from the original container, or from a container which has been prepared by a Florida licensed pharmacist. Only single doses of such preparations shall be removed from the container, and then only after the preparation has been prescribed for a specific patient, and the order has been duly recorded upon the records of the institution. This requirement shall not apply to nor be construed as preventing the administration of treatment in bona fide emergency cases, or further as prohibiting any person who is a duly licensed physician from dispensing medicinal drugs as defined in Chapter 465, F.S. A single dose of medicinal drugs based upon a valid physician's drug order may also be obtained and administered under the supervision of the nurse in charge consistent with good institutional practice procedures as established by the consultant pharmacist of record and written in the policy and procedure manual which shall be available within the pharmacy.
- A Class II institutional pharmacy may contract with a Special Parenteral/Enteral Extended Scope pharmacy for the pharmacy services provided for by Rule 64B16-28.860, F.A.C.

- Special Parenteral/Enteral Extended Scope pharmacies and institutional pharmacy permits shall create and comply with Policy and Procedure Manuals that delineate duties and responsibilities of each entity, including the following provisions:
    - The institutional pharmacy permit shall maintain records appropriate to ensure the provision of proper patient care.
    - The institutional pharmacy permit designee shall inspect and log in all medicinal drugs provided by the Special Parenteral/Enteral Extended Scope pharmacy.
    - A pharmacist for the institutional pharmacy shall provide drug utilization review and shall review each prescription order prior to transmission to the Special Parenteral/Enteral Extended Scope pharmacy.
- Such Policy and Procedure manuals shall be made available to the Board or Department upon request.
- Prior to contracting for such services the institutional pharmacy shall ensure that the Special Parenteral/Enteral Extended Scope pharmacy is licensed under the provisions of Rule 64B16-28.860, F.A.C.

Institutional Class II Pharmacy – Emergency Department Dispensing

- Individuals licensed to prescribe medicinal drugs in this state may dispense from the emergency department of a hospital holding a class II institutional pharmacy permit.
- The following records of prescribing and dispensing must be created by the prescriber/dispenser and maintained by the consultant pharmacist of record within the facility
    - Patient name and address

- Drug and strength prescribed/dispensed
- Quantity prescribed/dispensed
- Directions for use
- Prescriber/dispenser
- Prescriber DEA registration, if applicable.
- Reason community pharmacy services were not readily accessible.
- Must meet the prescription labeling requirements
- Quantity dispensed must not exceed a 24-hour supply or the minimal dispensable quantity, whichever is greater.

Class II Institutional Pharmacy Department Security

If there is not a pharmacist present and on duty then the pharmacy should be secured and no one can enter.

Class II Institutional Pharmacies – Automated Distribution and Packaging

Definitions
- "Automated medication system" means a robotic, mechanical or computerized device that is not used for medication compounding and is designed to:
  - Distribute medications in a licensed health care facility; or
  - Package medications for final distribution by a pharmacist.
- "Centralized automated medication system" means an automated medication system located in a pharmacy department from which medication is distributed or packaged for final distribution by a pharmacist.
- "Decentralized automated medication system" means an automated medication system that is located outside of a pharmacy department but within the same institution.
- "Distribute" or "Distribution" means the process of providing a drug to an individual authorized to administer medications and licensed as a health care

provider in the state of Florida pursuant to an order issued by an authorized prescriber.
- "Medication" means a medicinal drug or proprietary preparation.
- "Override medication" means a single dose of medication that may be removed from a decentralized automated medication system prior to pharmacist review because a practitioner licensed pursuant to Chapter 458, 459 or 466, F.S., determined that the clinical status of the patient would be significantly compromised by delay.
- "Low risk override medication" is a medication determined by a practitioner licensed pursuant to Chapters 458, 459, or 466, F.S., to have a low risk of drug allergy, drug interaction, dosing error, or adverse patient outcome, and may be removed from a decentralized automated medication system independent of a pharmacist's review of the medication order or clinical status of the patient.
- "Physician controlled medication" is medication distributed in an environment where a practitioner controls the order, preparation and administration of the medication.

General Requirements for the Use of Automated Medication Systems

- The consultant pharmacist of record shall be responsible for:
    o Maintaining a record of each transaction or operation;
    o Controlling access to the system;
    o Maintaining policies and procedures for;
        ▪ Operation of the automated medication system;
        ▪ Training personnel who use the automated medication system;
        ▪ Maintaining patient services whenever the automated medication system is not operating; and

- Defining a procedure for a pharmacist to grant or deny access to the medication in the system.
    - Security of the system;
    - Assuring that a patient receives the pharmacy services necessary for good pharmaceutical care in a timely manner;
    - Assuring that the system maintains the integrity of the information in the system and protects patient confidentiality;
    - Establishing a comprehensive Quality Assurance program;
    - Establishing a procedure for stocking or restocking the automated medication system; and
    - Ensuring compliance with all requirements for packaging and labeling.
- A pharmacist shall perform prospective drug use review and approve each medication order prior to administration of a medication except an override medication, a low risk override medication or a physician controlled medication.
- A pharmacist shall perform retrospective drug use review for an override medication.

<u>Multidisciplinary Committee for Decentralized Automated Medication Systems</u>
- The consultant pharmacist of record shall convene or identify a multidisciplinary committee, which is charged with oversight of the decentralized automated medication system.
- The Multidisciplinary Committee shall:
    - Include at least one pharmacist;
    - Establish the criteria and process for determining which medication qualifies as an override medication or a low risk override medication in a decentralized automated medication system;
    - Develop policies and procedures regarding the decentralized automated medication system; and

- - - o Have its decisions reviewed and approved by the consultant pharmacist of record.

Stocking or Restocking of a Decentralized Automated Medication System
- Medications in a decentralized Automated Medication System shall be stocked or restocked by a pharmacist, registered pharmacy intern, or by a registered pharmacy technician supervised by a pharmacist.
- The stocking or restocking of a decentralized automated medication system shall follow one of the following procedures to assure correct medication selection:
    - o A pharmacist shall conduct a daily audit of medications placed or to be placed into an automated medication system that includes random sampling.
    - o A bar code verification, electronic verification, or similar verification process shall be utilized to assure correct selection of medication placed or to be placed into an automated medication system. The utilization of a bar code, electronic, or similar verification technology shall require an initial quality assurance validation followed by a monthly quality assurance review by a pharmacist.

Centralized Automated Medication Systems. A pharmacist utilizing a centralized medication system may distribute patient specific medications within the licensed health care facility without checking each individual medication selected or packaged by the system, if:
- The initial medication order has been reviewed and approved by a pharmacist; and
- The medication is distributed for subsequent administration by a health care professional permitted by Florida law to administer medication; and
- A bar code verification, electronic verification, or similar verification process shall be utilized to assure correct selection of medication placed or to be placed into an

automated medication system. The utilization of a bar code, electronic verification, or similar verification technology shall require an initial quality assurance validation, followed by monthly quality assurance review by a pharmacist.

<u>Quality Assurance Program.</u> The consultant pharmacist of record shall be responsible for establishing a quality assurance program for the automated medication system. The program shall provide for:

- Review of override and low risk override medication utilization;
- Investigation of a medication error related to the automated medication system;
- Review of a discrepancy or transaction reports and identify patterns of inappropriate use or access;
- Review of the operation of the system;
- Integration of the automated medication system quality assurance program with the overall continuous quality improvement of the pharmacy as defined in Rule 64B16-27.300, F.A.C.; and
- Assurance that individuals working with the automated medication system receive appropriate training on the operation of the system and procedures for maintaining pharmacy services when the system is not in operation.

<u>Record Keeping</u>

- The consultant pharmacist of record shall maintain records related to the automated medication system in a readily retrievable manner.
- The following records shall be maintained for at least 60 days:
  - Daily audits of stocking or restocking, if applicable;
  - Daily audits for the output of centralized automated medication system, if applicable; and
  - Transaction records for all non-controlled medications or devices distributed by the automated medication system.

- The following records shall be maintained for at least two (2) years:
  - Any report or analysis generated as part of the quality assurance program;
  - A report or database related to access to the system or any change in the access to the system or to medication in the system; and
  - Transaction records from the automated medication system for all controlled substances dispensed or distributed.

Security. A decentralized automated medication system that contains controlled substances shall prohibit simultaneous access to multiple drug entities, drug strengths, or dosage forms of controlled substances, unless otherwise contained in labeled patient-specific form.

Remote Medication Order Processing for Class II Institutional Pharmacies

Definitions
- "Remote Medication Order Processing" includes any of the following activities performed for a Class II Institutional Pharmacy from a remote location:
  - Receiving, interpreting, or clarifying medication orders.
  - Entering or transferring medication order data.
  - Performing prospective drug use review.
  - Obtaining substitution authorizations.
  - Interpreting and acting on clinical data.
  - Performing therapeutic interventions.
  - Providing drug information.
  - Authorizing the release of a medication for administration.
- "Medication" means a medicinal drug or proprietary preparation.
- "Prospective drug use review" means an evaluation of medication orders and patient medication records for:
  - Over utilization or under utilization of medication.

- Therapeutic duplication of medication.
- Drug disease contraindications.
- Drug interactions.
- Incorrect drug dosage or duration of drug treatment.
- Clinical abuse or misuse of medication.

<u>General requirements</u>
- All pharmacists participating in remote medication order processing shall be Florida licensed pharmacists.
- Must have access to sufficient patient information necessary for prospective drug use review and approval of medication orders.
- A pharmacist shall perform the final check of a medication order.
- If the pharmacist performing remote order processing is not an employee of the Class II Institutional pharmacy, the Class II Institutional pharmacy must have a written agreement or contract with the pharmacist or entity employing the pharmacist. The written agreement or contract shall:
  - Outline the services to be provided.
  - Delineate the responsibilities of each party including compliance with federal and state laws and regulations governing the practice of pharmacy as well as state and federal medical privacy requirements.
  - Require that the parties adopt a policies and procedures manual.
  - Provide that the parties have access to or share a common electronic file such that the pharmacist performing remote medication order processing has sufficient patient information necessary for prospective drug use review and approval of medication orders.

<u>Policy and Procedures.</u> A policy and procedures manual shall:
- Be accessible to each party involved in remote medication order processing.

- Be available for inspection by the Board or an authorized agent of the Department.
- Outline the responsibilities of each party involved in remote medication order processing.
- Include a current list of the name, address, telephone number, and license number of each pharmacist involved in remote medication order processing.
- Include policies and procedures for:
  - Protecting the confidentiality and integrity of patient information.
  - Ensuring that a pharmacist performing prospective drug use review has access to appropriate drug information resources.
  - Ensuring that medical and nursing staff understand how to contact a pharmacist.
  - Maintaining records to identify the name, initials, or identification code of each person who performs a processing function for a medication order.
  - Complying with federal and state laws and regulations.
  - Operating or participating in a continuous quality improvement program for pharmacy services designed to objectively and systematically monitor and evaluate the quality and appropriateness of patient care, pursue opportunities to improve patient care, and resolve identified problems.
  - Reviewing the written policies and procedures and documenting the review every year.

<u>Records</u>
- A Class II Institutional Pharmacy involved in remote medication order processing shall maintain a record that identifies the name, initials, or identification code of each person who performed a processing function for every medication order. The record shall be available by medication order or by patient name.

- The record may be maintained in a common electronic file if the record is maintained in such a manner that the data processing system can produce a printout which identifies every person who performed a processing function for a medication order.
- The record shall be readily retrievable for at least the past two (2) years.
- The record shall be available for inspection by the Board or an authorized agent of the Department.

Automated Pharmacy System – Long Term Care, Hospice, and Prison
Definitions
- "Automated pharmacy system" means a mechanical system that performs operations or activities, other than compounding or administration, relative to the storage, packaging, counting, labeling, and delivery of a medicinal drug, and which collects, controls, and maintains a record of each transaction.
- "Provider pharmacy" means a pharmacy that provides pharmacy services by using an automated pharmacy system at a remote site.
- "Remote site" means a long term care facility or hospice, or a state correctional institution, that is not located at the same location as the provider pharmacy, at which pharmacy services are provided using an automated pharmacy system.
- "Controlled substance" means a substance listed in Chapter 893, F.S., or 21 CFR Part 1308.

Provider Pharmacy Requirements
- A provider pharmacy may provide pharmacy services to a long term care facility or hospice, or a state correctional institution, through the use of an automated pharmacy system.
- An automated pharmacy system shall only be used to provide pharmacy services to an inpatient or a resident of the remote site.

- Supervision of the automated pharmacy system shall be the responsibility of a Florida pharmacist employed by the provider pharmacy.
- Every medicinal drug stored in the automated pharmacy system shall be owned by the provider pharmacy.
- An automated pharmacy system shall be under the supervision of a pharmacist employed by the provider pharmacy. The pharmacist need not be physically present at the remote site if the system is supervised electronically.
- A provider pharmacy shall have policies and procedures to ensure adequate security.

<u>Prescription Department Manager Requirements</u>
- The prescription department manager shall ensure that the automated pharmacy system complies with Chapter 893, F.S., and 21 C.F.R., relating to the regulation of controlled substances, for each automated pharmacy system that contains a controlled substance.
- The prescription department manager shall ensure that the use of an automated pharmacy system does not compromise patient confidentiality.
- The prescription department manager or a designee shall:
    - Authorize or deny access to the data from an automated pharmacy system or to a drug stored inside the automated pharmacy system.
    - Document the training of each person who has access to the data from an automated pharmacy system or to a drug stored inside the automated pharmacy system.

<u>Automated Pharmacy System Requirements</u>
- A medicinal drug stored in bulk or unit-of-use in an automated pharmacy system is part of the inventory of the provider pharmacy and is not part of the inventory of any other pharmacy permit for the facility.
- A medicinal drug may be removed from an automated pharmacy system for administration to a patient only

after a prescription or order has been received and approved by a pharmacist at the provider pharmacy. This provision does not apply to a medication designated as an emergency medication if the automated pharmacy system is also used as an emergency medication kit in compliance with Section 400.142, F.S. and Rule 59A-4.112, F.A.C.
- A pharmacist at the provider pharmacy shall control all operations of the automated pharmacy system and approve release of the initial dose of a prescription or order. A subsequent dose from an approved prescription or order may be released without additional approval of a pharmacist. However, any change made in a prescription or order shall require a new approval by a pharmacist to release the drug.
- A pharmacist at the provider pharmacy shall comply with the patient record requirements in Rule 64B16-27.800, F.A.C., and prospective drug use review requirements in Rule 64B16-27.810, F.A.C., for every medicinal drug delivered through an automated pharmacy system.
- If the facility where pharmacy services are being provided maintains a medication administration record that includes directions for use of the medication, a unit dose medication may be utilized if the provider pharmacy or the automated pharmacy system identifies and records the dispensing pharmacy, the prescription or order number, the name of the patient, and the name of the prescribing practitioner for each medicinal drug delivered.
- Stocking or Restocking of an Automated Pharmacy System.
    - The stocking or restocking of a medicinal drug in an automated pharmacy system at the remote site shall be completed by a pharmacist or other licensed personnel, except as provided in the subparagraph below of this section.

- o If the automated pharmacy system uses removable cartridges or containers to store the drug, the stocking or restocking of the cartridges or containers may occur at the provider pharmacy and be sent to the remote site to be loaded by personnel designated by the pharmacist if:
  - A pharmacist verifies the cartridge or container has been properly filled and labeled.
  - The individual cartridge or container is transported to the remote site in a secure, tamper-evident container.
  - The automated pharmacy system uses bar code verification, electronic verification, or similar process to assure that the cartridge or container is accurately loaded into the automated pharmacy system.
- A medicinal drug that has been removed from the automated pharmacy system shall not be replaced into the system unless a pharmacist has examined the medication, the packaging, and the labeling and determined that reuse of the medication is appropriate.
- Medication to be returned to the provider pharmacy's stock shall meet the requirements of Rule 64B16-28.118, F.A.C.

Security Requirements
- If a provider pharmacy intends to store a controlled substance in an automated pharmacy system:
  - o It shall maintain a separate DEA registration for each remote site at which a controlled substance is stored.
  - o It may utilize one DEA registration to include multiple automated pharmacy systems located at a single address.
- A provider pharmacy shall only store a medicinal drug at a remote site within an automated pharmacy system

- which is locked by a mechanism that prevents access to a drug or to data by unauthorized personnel.
- Access to the drugs shall be limited to a pharmacist or a registered pharmacy technician employed by the provider pharmacy or licensed personnel in the facility or institution who are authorized to administer medication.
- An automated pharmacy system that contains a controlled substance shall prohibit simultaneous access to multiple drug entities, drug strengths, or dosage forms of controlled substances.

Emergency medication. If an automated pharmacy system is utilized for both a medication ordered for a specific patient and an emergency medication for which the review of a pharmacist is not required:
- The emergency medication shall be stored separately from other patient medications.
- The record shall identify the storage location from which the medication was released.
- The record shall include the name of the medication, the patient, the prescriber, the person who accessed the automated pharmacy system, and the date and time of the release.

Record Keeping Requirements
- The record of transactions with the automated pharmacy system shall be maintained in a readily retrievable manner.
- The record shall be available to an authorized agent of the Department of Health or the Board of Pharmacy.
- The record shall include:
    - Name or identification of the patient or resident.
    - Name, strength and dosage form of the drug product released.
    - Quantity of drug released.
    - Date and time of each release of a drug.
    - Name of provider pharmacy.
    - Prescription number or order number.
    - Name of prescribing practitioner.

- o Identity of the pharmacist who approved the prescription or order.
- o Identity of the person to whom the drug was released.
- A record of every transaction with the automated pharmacy system shall be maintained for two (2) years.

Modified Class II Institutional Pharmacies
- Modified Class II Institutional Pharmacies are those Institutional Pharmacies which provide specialized pharmacy services restricted in scope of practice and designed to provide certain health care pharmacy services that are not generally obtainable from other pharmacy permittees. These specialized institutional pharmacy practices are generally identifiable with short-term or primary care treatment modalities in entities such as primary alcoholism treatment centers, free-standing emergency rooms, rapid in/out surgical centers, certain county health programs, and correctional institutions. Medicinal drugs may not be administered, except to patients of the institution for use on the premises of the institution, in any facility which has been issued a Modified Class II Institutional Pharmacy Permit. All medicinal drugs as defined by Section 465.003(7), F.S., which are stocked in these pharmacies are only to be administered on premises as defined by Section 465.003(1), F.S., to inpatients on an inpatient or in-program basis. In-program patients are defined as those patients who have met program admission criteria required by the institution.
- Modified Class II Institutional Pharmacies are categorized according to the type of specialized pharmaceutical delivery system utilized and the following criteria (Categories are designated as Type "A", Type "B" and Type "C"):
    - o The type of the medicinal drug delivery system utilized at the facility, either a patient-specific or

bulk drug system, and, the quantity of the medicinal drug formulary at the facility,
- Type "A" Modified Class II Institutional Pharmacies provide pharmacy services in a facility which has a formulary of not more than 15 medicinal drugs, excluding those medicinal drugs contained in an emergency box, and in which the medicinal drugs are stored in bulk and in which the consultant pharmacist shall provide on-site consultations not less than once every month, unless otherwise directed by the Board after review of the policy and procedure manual.
- Type "B" Modified Class II Institutional Pharmacies provide pharmacy services in a facility in which medicinal drugs are stored in the facility in patient specific form and in bulk form and which has an expanded drug formulary, and in which the consultant pharmacist shall provide on-site consultations not less than once per month, unless otherwise directed by the Board after review of the policy and procedure manual.
- Type "C" Modified Class II Institutional Pharmacies provide pharmacy services in a facility in which medicinal drugs are stored in the facility in patient specific form and which has an expanded drug formulary, and in which the consultant pharmacist shall provide on-site consultations not less than once per month, unless otherwise directed by the Board after review of the policy and procedure manual.
- All Modified Class II Institutional Pharmacies shall be under the control and supervision of a certified consultant pharmacist.
- The consultant pharmacist of record for the Modified Class II Institutional Pharmacy shall be responsible for establishing a written protocol and a policy and procedure manual for the implementation of a drug

delivery system to be utilized and the requirements of this rule.
- A copy of the permittee's policy and procedure manual as provided herein shall accompany the permit application. The original policy and procedure manual shall be kept within the Modified Class II Institutional Pharmacy and shall be available for inspection by the Department of Health.
- Drugs stocked in Modified Class II Institutional Pharmacies, Type "A" and Type "B" as provided herein, shall be those drugs generally utilized in the treatment modalities encompassed within the health care scope of the particular institutional care entity. The protocol and the policy and procedure manual for Type "A" and Type "B" Modified Class II Institutional Pharmacies shall contain definitive information as to drugs and strengths thereof to be stocked.
    - The policy and procedure manual of facilities which are issued Type A Modified Class II Institutional Permits shall provide the following:
        - Definitive information as to drugs and strengths to be stored.
        - The establishment of a Pharmacy Services Committee which shall meet at least annually.
        - Provisions for the handling of the emergency box including the utilization of separate logs for recordkeeping.
        - Provisions for the secure ordering, storage and recordkeeping of all medicinal drugs at the facility.
        - Provisions for the utilization of proof-of-use forms for all medicinal drugs within the facility.
        - A diagram of the facility and the security and storage of the medicinal drugs.

- Provisions for maintaining the records of consultations for not less than two (2) years at the facility which shall be stored on-site and available for inspection by the Department of Health.
  - The policy and procedure manual of facilities which are issued Type B Modified Class II Institutional Permits shall provide the following:
    - The establishment of a Pharmacy Services Committee which shall meet at least annually.
    - Provisions for the handling of the emergency box including the utilization of separate logs for recordkeeping.
    - Provisions for the secure ordering, storage and recordkeeping of all medicinal drugs at the facility.
    - Provisions for the utilization of a perpetual inventory system for all controlled substances, injectables and other medicinal drugs as required by the Pharmacy Services Committee.
    - A diagram of the facility and the security and storage of the medicinal drugs.
    - Provisions for maintaining the records of consultations for not less than two (2) years at the facility which shall be stored on-site and available for inspection by the Department of Health.
  - The policy and procedure manual of facilities which are issued Type C Modified Class II Institutional Permit shall provide the following:
    - The establishment of a Pharmacy Services Committee which shall meet at least annually.

- - Provisions for the handling of the emergency box including the utilization of separate logs for recordkeeping.
  - Provisions for the secure ordering, storage and recordkeeping of all medicinal drugs at the facility.
  - Provisions for the utilization of a Medication Administration Record (MAR) for all medicinal drugs administered to patients of the facility.
  - A diagram of the facility and the security and storage of the medicinal drugs.
  - Provisions for maintaining the records of consultations for not less than two (2) years at the facility which shall be stored on-site and available for inspection by the Department of Health.
- Controlled drugs stocked as provided herein within a Type "A" Modified Class II Institutional Pharmacy shall be stocked in unit size not to exceed 100 dosage units unless an exception thereto is granted by the Board of Pharmacy. Proof of use record sheets showing patient's name, date of administration, initials of person administering drug, and other pertinent control requirements are required for both controlled and noncontrolled substance medicinal drugs in Type "A" Modified Class II Institutional Pharmacies.
- A Modified Class II institutional pharmacy may contract with a Special Parenteral/Enteral Extended Scope pharmacy for the pharmacy services provided for by Rule 64B16-28.860, F.A.C.
  - Special Parenteral/Enteral Extended Scope pharmacies and institutional pharmacy permits shall create and comply with Policy and Procedure Manuals that delineate duties and responsibilities of each entity including the following provisions:

- - The institutional pharmacy permit shall maintain records appropriate to ensure the provision of proper patient care.
  - The institutional pharmacy permit designee shall inspect and log in all medicinal drugs provided by the Special Parenteral/Enteral Extended Scope pharmacy.
  - Such Policy and Procedure manuals shall be made available to the Board or Department upon request.
  - Prior to contracting for such services the institutional pharmacy shall ensure that the Special Parenteral/Enteral Extended Scope pharmacy is licensed under the provisions of Rule 64B16-28.860, F.A.C.

Special Pharmacies

- Special pharmacies are pharmacies providing miscellaneous specialized pharmacy service functions. The Board of Pharmacy, by this rule, provides for the establishment of the following special pharmacy permits:
  - Special-Limited Community.
  - Special-Parenteral and Enteral.
  - Special-Closed System Pharmacy.
  - Special-Non Resident (Mail Service).
  - Special-End Stage Renal Disease.
  - Special-Parenteral/Enteral Extended Scope.
  - Special-ALF.
- An applicant for any special pharmacy permit shall provide the Board of Pharmacy with an application (Form DOH\PH105 Revised 7/23/98, effective 11/11/98, which is hereby incorporated by reference and which can be obtained from the Department of Health) and a Policy and Procedure Manual which sets forth a detailed description of the type of pharmacy services to be provided within the special pharmacy

practice. The Policy and Procedure Manual shall contain detailed provisions for compliance with the provision of Section 465.0196, F.S., and other applicable requirements contained in this chapter.
- The Policy and Procedure Manual shall be prepared, maintained, and will be reviewed and is subject to approval by the Board of Pharmacy or its designee prior to the issuance of the permit and the initiation of the operation of the permittee. The policy and procedure manual is reviewed to determine if the operation of the facility will be in compliance with Chapters 465 and 893, F.S., and Chapter 64B16, F.A.C. The Policy and Procedure Manual shall be made available upon request of the Board or its agents. The applicant who requests a special permit shall be subject to inspection prior to the issuance of the permit.

Special Pharmacy – Limited Community Permit

A Special-Limited Community Permit shall be obtained by a Class II Institutional Pharmacy that dispenses medicinal drugs, including controlled substances to:
- Employees, medical staff and their dependents for their personal use,
- Patients of the hospital who are under a continuation of a course of therapy not to exceed a three (3) day supply,
- Patients obtaining medical services in the facility's emergency room and, whenever it is otherwise appropriate, as indicated in the applicant's policy and procedure manual.

Sterile Products and Special Parenteral/Enteral Compounding

Sterile Products and Parenteral/Enteral Compounding.
- A sterile products and parenteral/enteral compounding pharmacy is a type of special pharmacy as provided by Section 465.0196, F.S., which is limited in scope of pharmacy practice to render sterile products and

parenteral/enteral compounding functions. This pharmacy practice facilitates the utilization of certain institutional therapeutic measures by patients in the home environment or by patients in an institutional environment where such pharmacy service is unavailable. Pharmacy services, sterile products and parenteral/enteral products provided by a special sterile products and parenteral/enteral compounding pharmacy pursuant to prescription as defined by Section 465.003(13), F.S., shall be limited to the compounding and/or dispensing of:
  - Sterile preparations for parenteral therapy, parenteral nutrition, and/or
  - Sterile preparations for jejunostomy feeding and sterile irrigation solutions, and/or
  - Sterile preparations of cytotoxic or antineo-plastic agents, and/or
  - Sterile products (i.e., injectables, eye drops, etc.).
- Prior to engaging in a sterile products and parenteral/enteral compounding pharmacy practice an entity shall obtain a special sterile products and parenteral/enteral compounding pharmacy permit as provided herein.

<u>Pharmacy Environment.</u> The compounding and dispensing of sterile products and parenteral/enteral prescription preparations within a special sterile products and parenteral/enteral compounding pharmacy shall be accomplished in a pharmacy environment subject to the pharmacy permit laws of this state and in accordance with those requirements for the safe handling of drugs. The environment for this practice shall be set apart, and designed, and equipped to facilitate controlled aseptic conditions. Aseptic techniques shall prevail in this practice to minimize the possibility of microbial contamination.

<u>General Requirements.</u>
- A special sterile products and parenteral/enteral compounding pharmacy shall be under the control and

supervision of a licensed pharmacist, who shall be designated prescription department manager on the application for a special sterile products and parenteral/enteral compounding pharmacy. The prescription department manager or other licensed qualified pharmacist as provided herein shall be present on duty during all hours of operation of said pharmacy. Changes in prescription department manager shall be reported to the Board of Pharmacy office within 10 days by the permit holder and prescription department manager of record. A prescription department manager of a special sterile products and parenteral/enteral compounding pharmacy shall not be designated prescription department manager of record of more than one special sterile products and parenteral/enteral compounding pharmacy, unless otherwise approved by the Board. The Board will consider the proximity of the facility as well as the administrative workload created by the two permits, in determining whether or not it will approve the designation of someone as a prescription department manager of more than one special sterile products and parenteral/enteral compounding pharmacy.

- A special sterile products and parenteral/enteral compounding pharmacy shall provide special handling and packaging of compounded parenteral and enteral preparations when delivering from the pharmacy to the patient or institution as required to maintain stability of the preparations. All such preparations shall include the time and/or date of expiration on the label. Delivery from the pharmacy to the patient shall be made within a reasonable time. A special sterile products and parenteral/enteral compounding pharmacy shall provide telephone accessibility to its pharmacist(s) for its patients at all hours.
- A patient profile shall be maintained for each patient. The profile must contain available medical information

consistent with prevailing pharmacy standards which shall be confidential.
- A Policy and Procedure Manual shall be prepared and maintained at each special sterile products and parenteral/enteral compounding pharmacy, and be available for inspection by authorized agents of the Board of Pharmacy and the Department. The Policy and Procedure Manual shall set forth in detail the objectives and operational guidelines of the permittee. The Policy and Procedure Manual shall include a Quality Assurance Program which monitors personnel qualifications, training and performance, equipment facilities, and random production sampling consistent with recommended standards for compounding and dispensing intravenous admixtures as set forth by the Joint Commission on Accreditation of Health Organizations, the National Coordinating Committee and Large Volume Parenteral, and as provided by the Florida Board of Pharmacy.
- Compounding shall be conducted within an annually certified laminar air flow (LAF) hood, except in the existence of a Class 100 certified compounding environment, or certified mobile isolation chamber, in which case compounding may be conducted without the use of a certified laminar air flow hood. All cytotoxins must be compounded in a certified vertical laminar air flow hood or certified mobile isolation chamber. The use of a Type A or Type B LAF hood used shall be dependent upon the volume of work anticipated. All certifications shall be performed following manufacturer specification.
- Protective garb: gloves, face and eye, and gowns should be provided and used.
- Proper aseptic procedures must be used at all times to prevent bacterial contamination of the product as well as chemical contamination of the operator.

- All unused cytotoxic agents and material must be disposed of properly in accordance with accepted professional standards and applicable law.

Minimum Requirements for Space, Equipment, Supplies and Publications

- To ensure compliance with the general requirements as set forth, the following minimum requirements for space, equipment, supplies and publications shall be met by a pharmacy which operates under the special permit of a sterile products and parenteral/enteral compounding pharmacy. These requirements are in addition to the minimum requirements for space and equipment required of other types of pharmacies when applicable. The minimum permit requirements are set forth as follows:
- Space:
    - The area for preparing sterile prescriptions as provided for by this rule referred to as the sterile admixture room shall be set apart from general work and storage areas. The room shall be adequately air conditioned or shall be under positive pressure.
    - The sterile admixture room shall provide space for a minimum of one laminar flow hood. Additionally, the space shall be of adequate size to accommodate other equipment as provided herein and sufficient space to allow pharmacists and other employees working therein to adequately, safely, and accurately fulfill their duties related to prescriptions.
- Equipment:
    - Laminar Air Flow Hood(s):
        - Horizontal and/or.
        - Vertical.
    - Refrigerator/freezer convenient to the clean room.
    - Sink and wash area convenient to the clean room.

- - Appropriate waste containers for:
    - Used needles and syringes.
    - All cytotoxic waste including apparel.
- Supplies:
  - Gloves, masks and gowns.
  - Needles and syringes of various standard sizes.
  - Disinfectant cleaning agents.
  - Clean towels.
  - Handwashing materials with bactericidal properties.
  - Vacuum containers and various transfer sets.
  - "Spill kits" for cytotoxic agent spills.
- Current References:
  - Chapter 465, F.S.
  - Chapter 499, F.S.
  - Chapter 893, F.S.
  - Title 64B16, F.A.C., Rules of the Florida Board of Pharmacy.
  - United States Pharmacopeia and National Formulary, or Remington Pharmaceutical Sciences, or the United States Dispensatory (along with the latest supplements), or an equivalent thereof sufficient in scope to meet the professional practice needs of the pharmacy, and a current authoritative therapeutic reference.
  - Handbook of Injectable Drugs by American Society of Hospital Pharmacists.
  - "Practice Guidelines For Personnel Dealing With Cytotoxic Drugs."

A community pharmacy permittee may perform parenteral/enteral compounding or prepare sterile products without obtaining an additional permit under this section, so long as prior to entering into such activities, the community pharmacy meets the requirements of subsections (1)-(5) above and is inspected for compliance by the Department of Health.

Special – Closed System Pharmacy

- A Special – Closed System Pharmacy permit is a type of special pharmacy as provided for by Section 465.0196, F.S., which dispenses medicinal drugs, utilizing closed delivery systems, to facilities where prescriptions are individually prepared for the ultimate consumer, including nursing homes, jails, ALF's (Adult Congregate Living Facilities), ICF-MR's (Intermediate Care Facility/Mentally Retarded) or other custodial care facilities when defined by AHCA rules which the Board may approve.
- A special – closed system pharmacy permittee shall maintain a policy and procedure manual including drug procurement, storage, handling, compounding, dispensing, record keeping and disposition.
- A special – closed system pharmacy permittee shall provide twenty-four hour emergency and on-call service.
- A special – closed system pharmacy permittee may dispense parenteral and enteral medications as provided by rule.
- A special – closed system pharmacy permittee shall be under the supervision of a prescription department manager who is responsible for maintaining all drug records, providing security of the prescription department and following other rules as relate to the practice of pharmacy. The prescription department manager of a closed system pharmacy shall not be the prescription department manager of any other pharmacy permit except when the permit is within the premises of a community pharmacy permit.
- The utilization of registered pharmacy interns and registered pharmacy technicians is subject to the rules as provided by Rule 64B16-26.400, F.A.C.

Special – Non Resident (Mail Service)

- A Special – Non Resident (Mail Service) pharmacy is located outside this state delivering a dispensed medicinal drug in any manner into this state.
- The pharmacy and the pharmacist designated as the prescription department manager or equivalent, for dispensing into Florida, must be licensed in the state of location.
- Changes of location, corporate officers, and prescription department managers must be reported to the Board.
- The pharmacy must have regular hours of operation of not less than six (6) days per week and not less than forty (40) hours per week. A toll-free telephone number must be available to patients.
- A pharmacy outside of this state and not registered as a Non Resident Pharmacy may make a one-time delivery of a dispensed medicinal drug to a patient in this state.

Special Pharmacy – ESRD

An ESRD Pharmacy is a type of special pharmacy which is limited in scope of pharmacy practice to the provision of dialysis products and supplies to persons with chronic kidney failure for self-administration at the person's home or specified address. Pharmacy services and dialysis supplies and products provided by an ESRD pharmacy shall be limited to the distribution and delivery of legend drugs and devices included below; which are ordered by a physician for administration or delivery to a person with chronic kidney failure for self-administration at the person's home or specified address.

- Schedule of legend drugs:
    - Saline Solutions
    - Porcine Heparin
    - Beef Heparin
    - Dextrose Solutions
    - Doxercalciferol
    - Epoetin Alfa
    - NACL INJ 50 MEQ/20 ML

- o Levocarnitine
- o Lidocaine
- o Vitamin Preparations (dialysate use only)
- o Paricalcitrol
- o Peritoneal Dialysate Solutions
- o Protamine Sulfate
- o Potassium 20 MEQ/10ML (dialysate use only)
- o Sodium Ferric Gluconate Complex or equivalent
- o Sterile Water for Irrigation.
- The schedule of legend devices includes:
  - o Hemodialyzers
  - o Hemodialysis solutions
  - o Bloodlines and Associated Connectology
  - o Peritoneal Dialysis Tubing and Connectology
- The provision of legend drugs and devices included in the schedule necessary to perform dialysis to a person with chronic kidney failure for self-administration at the person's home or specified address shall be under the professional supervision of an appropriate practitioner licensed under Florida law. The consultant pharmacist shall assure that the following occurs:
  - o Prescription required for any legend drugs and/or devices
  - o Person with chronic kidney failure has been trained (documentation necessary) in the proper use and administration
- The ESRD pharmacy shall deliver products to a person with chronic kidney failure only upon receipt of a valid prescription from a prescribing practitioner specifying or including:
  - o Documentation that the intended recipient of the products has been trained in home dialysis therapy and will require such products
  - o The duration of prescribing practitioner's order; and
  - o The name and product code of each product prescribed and the quantity prescribed.

- - The prescription may indicate the person with chronic kidney failure shall have the right to request refills of legend drugs, devices or both, included in the schedule and described in the order for a period of one year.
- Labeling requirements and must be inspected by the consulting pharmacist or 2 trained employees:
  - "Use as Directed" statement
  - The name and address of the person to whom the products will be delivered
  - The name of the prescribing practitioner
  - The name and address of the ESRD pharmacy location from which the products were shipped
  - The prescription number identifying the shipment to the order created by the prescribing practitioner; and
  - Any special instructions regarding delivery dates or locations
  - The date after which the drug(s) and/or device(s) must be discarded. Notwithstanding any other rule, the ESRD pharmacy may use, in lieu of a discard after date, the manufactures expiration date when such is displayed in an unopened sealed package.
- In addition to the foregoing operation requirements, an ESRD pharmacy shall comply with the following:
  - The ESRD pharmacy license shall be displayed at each ESRD pharmacy location
  - The Board of Pharmacy shall be notified in writing of the Consulting Pharmacist responsible, at the time of application for the permit, for supervising the ESRD pharmacy operations and within 10 days, if the Consultant Pharmacist of record changes.
  - The ESRD pharmacy's hours of business shall be posted. The ESRD pharmacy shall be open such hours as are necessary to safely and effectively

dispense and deliver supplies to those persons designated by the applicable prescribing practitioner. An ESRD pharmacy shall provide twenty-four hour emergency and on-call service.
    o The ESRD pharmacy shall maintain a current copy of the Florida pharmacy laws and rules.
- An ESRD pharmacy shall be under the control and supervision of licensed Consultant Pharmacist licensed under Section 465.0125, F.S. The Consulting Pharmacist shall be responsible for the drug/device delivery system.
- The Consultant Pharmacist of record for the ESRD Pharmacy shall be responsible for establishing a written protocol and Policy and Procedure Manual for the implementation of a delivery system to be utilized in compliance with the requirements of this Rule.
- The Consultant Pharmacist shall inspect the permitted ESRD pharmacy on a monthly basis.

Special Pharmacy – Parenteral/Enteral Extended Scope Permit
- A Special Parenteral/Enteral Extended Scope permit, as authorized by Section 465.0196, F.S., is required for pharmacies to compound patient specific enteral/parenteral preparations in conjunction with institutional pharmacy permits, provided requirements set forth herein are satisfied. Prior to engaging in a parenteral/enteral compounding pharmacy practice as described in this section, an entity shall obtain a Special Parenteral/Enteral Extended Scope pharmacy permit.
- Special Parenteral/Enteral Extended Scope pharmacies and institutional pharmacy permits shall create and comply with Policy and Procedure Manuals that delineate duties and responsibilities of each entity, including the following provisions:
    o When dispensing patient specific prescriptions provided by an institutional pharmacy permit, the Special Parenteral/Enteral Extended Scope

pharmacy shall confirm accuracy of the prescription and dosage.
    - The institutional pharmacy permit shall maintain records appropriate to ensure the provision of proper patient care.
    - The institutional pharmacy permit designee shall inspect and log in all medicinal drugs provided by the Special Parenteral/Enteral Extended Scope pharmacy.
    - A pharmacist for the Class II institutional pharmacy shall provide drug utilization review and shall review each prescription order prior to transmission to the Special Parenteral/Enteral Extended Scope pharmacy.
    - The Policy and Procedure Manual for a Special Parenteral/Enteral Extended Scope pharmacy shall also meet the policy and procedure manual requirements of paragraph 64B16-28.820(3)(d), F.A.C.
- Facilities obtaining this permit may also provide services described in paragraph 64B16-28.820(1)(a), F.A.C., without obtaining an additional permit. Pharmacy services and parenteral/enteral products provided by a Special Parenteral/Enteral Extended Scope pharmacy shall be limited to the compounding and/or dispensing of sterile:
    - Preparations for parental therapy, parenteral nutrition, and/or
    - Preparations for enteral feeding and sterile irrigation solutions, and/or
    - Preparations of cytotoxic or antineoplastic agents.
- Facilities operating under this permit may provide all necessary supplies and delivery systems so that the medicinal drugs listed herein may be properly administered.
- Pharmacy Environment. The compounding and dispensing of sterile parenteral/enteral prescription

preparations within a Special Parenteral/Enteral Extended Scope pharmacy shall be accomplished in a pharmacy environment subject to the pharmacy permit laws contained in Chapter 465, F.S., and in accordance with those requirements for the safe handling of drugs. Special Parenteral/Enteral Extended Scope permittees shall comply with the requirements contained in subsections 64B16-28.820(3) through (4), F.A.C., and the following:
- Shall include an active and ongoing end product testing program to ensure stability, sterility, and quantitative integrity of finished prescriptions.
- Shall insure each compounding process undergoes an initial and thereafter annual sterility validation utilizing media fill to ensure the integrity and validity of the compounding process.

- Records.
  - Special Parenteral/Enteral Extended Scope pharmacies shall comply with the record maintenance requirements as contained in Rule 64B16-28.140, F.A.C.
  - Special Parenteral/Enteral Extended Scope pharmacies dispensing medicinal products to patients under the provisions of paragraph 64B16-28.820(1)(a), F.A.C., or to patients of Modified Class II institutional pharmacies under the provisions of Rule 64B16-28.860, F.A.C., shall comply with the records, utilization review, and patient counseling requirements of Rules 64B16-27.800, 64B16-27.810 and 64B16-27.820, F.A.C.
  - Special Parenteral/Enteral Extended Scope pharmacies dispensing medicinal products to patients of Class II institutional pharmacies under the provisions of Rule 64B16-28.860, F.A.C., shall be exempt from the records, utilization review, and patient counseling requirements of Rules

64B16-27.800, 64B16-27.810 and 64B16-27.820, F.A.C.
- Compounding records shall be organized in such a manner as to include: lot number traceability of components used during compounding, documentation of any equipment used during compounding, documentation of staff performing compounding, and records recording ultimate dispensing of the compounded product.

Special-ALF

The Special-ALF permit is an optional facility license for those Assisted Living Facilities providing a drug delivery system utilizing medicinal drugs provided in unit dose packaging
- All medicinal drugs must be maintained in individual prescription containers for the individual patient
- Medicinal drugs may not be dispensed on the premises.
- Medicinal drugs dispensed to patients of Special-ALF permits may be returned to the dispensing pharmacy's stock under the provisions of Rule 64B16-28.118, F.A.C.
- Dispensed controlled substances that have been discontinued shall be disposed of under the provisions of Rule 64B16-28.301, F.A.C.
- Medicinal drugs dispensed to the residents of a Special-ALF permit shall meet the labeling requirements of Rule 64B16-28.502 and paragraph 64B16-28.402(1)(h), F.A.C.
- Each facility holding a Special-ALF permit shall designate a consultant pharmacist of record to ensure compliance with the laws and rules governing the permit.
- The Board office shall be notified in writing within 10 days of any change in the consultant pharmacist of record.
- The consultant pharmacist of record shall be responsible for the preparation of the Policy and Procedure Manual required by subsection 64B16-28.800(2), F.A.C. Policy and Procedure Manuals must provide for the appropriate

storage conditions and security of the medicinal drugs stored at the facility.
- The consultant pharmacist of record shall inspect the facility and prepare a written report to be filed at the permitted facility at least monthly.

Definitions – Nuclear Pharmacy

- A "nuclear pharmacy" is a pharmacy which provides radiopharmaceutical services.
- A "nuclear pharmacist" is a pharmacist who has met the training qualifications as described in Rule 64B16-28.903, F.A.C., and has been licensed by the Board of Pharmacy.
- A "radiopharmaceutical service" shall include, but shall not be limited to, the procurement, storage, preparation, labeling, quality assurance testing, distribution, record keeping and disposal of radiopharmaceuticals.
- A "radiopharmaceutical" is any substance defined as a drug by section 201(g)(1) of the Federal Food, Drug and Cosmetic Act which exhibits spontaneous disintegration of unstable nuclei with the emission of nuclear particles or photons and includes any such drug which is intended to be made radioactive. This definition includes nonradioactive reagent kits and nuclide generators which are intended to be used in the preparation of any such substance but does not include drugs such as carbon-containing compounds or potassium-containing salts which contain trace quantities of naturally occurring radionuclides.
- "Radiopharmaceutical quality assurance" includes, but is not limited to, the performance of appropriate chemical, biological and physical tests on radiopharmaceuticals, and the interpretation of the resulting data to determine their suitability for use in humans and animals, including internal test assessment, authentication of product history and the keeping of proper records.

- "Authentication of product history" includes, but is not limited to, identifying the purchasing source, the ultimate fate, and intermediate handling of any component of a radiopharmaceutical or other drug.

Nuclear Pharmacy – General Requirements

The process employed by any permit holder in this state concerning the handling of radioactive materials must involve appropriate procedures for the purchase, receipt, storage, manipulation, compounding, distribution and disposal of radioactive materials. In order to insure the public health and safety in this respect, a nuclear pharmacy in this state shall meet the following general requirements:

- Each nuclear pharmacy shall designate a nuclear pharmacist as the prescription department manager who shall be responsible for compliance with all laws and regulations, both state and federal pertaining to radiopharmaceuticals and radiopharmaceutical services. A nuclear pharmacist must personally supervise the operation of only one nuclear pharmacy during all times when radiopharmaceutical services are being performed.
- The nuclear pharmacy area shall be secured from access by unauthorized personnel.
- Each nuclear pharmacy shall maintain accurate records of the acquisition, inventory, distribution, and disposal of all radiopharmaceuticals.
- All nuclear pharmacies shall provide a secured radioactive storage and decay area.
- Nuclear pharmacies shall comply with all applicable laws and regulations of federal and state agencies for the procurement, secure storage, inventory, preparation, distribution and disposal of radiopharmaceuticals and other drugs.
- Radiopharmaceuticals are to be distributed only upon a prescription order from an authorized licensed medical practitioner or through the practitioner's agent.

- A nuclear pharmacist may transfer radioactive materials in accordance with all applicable laws and regulations.
- A nuclear pharmacist upon receiving an oral prescription order for a radiopharmaceutical shall immediately have the prescription order reduced to writing. The pharmacist may delegate this duty to a registered pharmacy technician. The prescription order shall contain at least the following:
    - The name of the user or his agent
    - The date of distribution and the time of administration of the radiopharmaceutical
    - The name of the procedure
    - The name of the radiopharmaceutical
    - The dose or quantity of the radiopharmaceutical
    - The serial number assigned to the prescription order for the radiopharmaceutical
    - Any specific instructions
    - The initials of the person who received the prescription order
    - The patient's name must be obtained and recorded prior to dispensing, if the prescription order is for a therapeutic or blood product radiopharmaceutical.
- The immediate outer container shield of a radiopharmaceutical to be dispensed shall be labeled with:
    - The name of and address of the pharmacy
    - The name of the prescriber
    - The date of the original filling
    - The standard radiation symbol
    - The words "Caution Radioactive Material"
    - The name of the procedure
    - The prescription order number of the radiopharmaceutical
    - The radionuclide and chemical form
    - The amount of radioactivity and the calibration date and time

- The expiration date and time
- The volume if a liquid
- The number of items or weight, if a solid
- The number of ampules or vials, if a gas
- Molybdenum 99 content to USP limits, applies only to TC 99M products
- The name of the patient or the words "Physician's Use Only" in the absence of a patient name. If the prescription order is for a therapeutic or blood-product radiopharmaceutical, the patient's name must be obtained and recorded prior to dispensing. The requirements of this subsection shall be met when the name of the patient is readily retrievable from the physician upon demand.
- The initials of the pharmacist who dispensed the medication.
- The immediate inner container label of a radiopharmaceutical to be distributed shall be labeled with:
  - The standard radiation symbol
  - The words "Caution Radioactive Material"
  - The radionuclide
  - The chemical form
  - The prescription order number of the radiopharmaceutical

Nuclear Pharmacy – Minimum Requirements

There are minimum requirements in addition to the general safety requirements for the control of radiation hazards. See the law for more information.

Animal Control Shelter Permits

An "animal control shelter" is a county or municipal animal control agency or Humane Society registered with the Secretary of State which holds a modified Class II Institutional Pharmacy permit issued by the Department of Health. An animal control shelter is issued a pharmacy permit for the sole purpose of obtaining the drugs, sodium pentobarbital and sodium pentobarbital with lidocaine, for euthanization of animals.

- Biennial permit
- Must apply to the DEA as well
- Consultant pharmacist requirement not necessary
- Sodium pentobarbital and sodium pentobarbital with lidocaine must be kept in a securely locked cabinet within a locked storage room.
- Schedule II order forms must be kept in a securely locked cabinet within a locked storage room.
- License can be suspended if terminated from or failing to successfully complete an impaired practitioners treatment program.
- License can be suspended or put on probation if test positive for any drug on any confirmed pre-employment or employer ordered drug screening when the practitioner does not have a lawful prescription and legitimate medical reason for using such drug.
- Information required on controlled substance prescriptions: practitioner's address, practitioner's DEA registration number, patient's address.
- Dispensing pharmacists must certify the daily hard-copy printout or daily log
- If licensee fails to complete the continuing education requirements in the biennial period, then they are required to take two additional hours of continuing education for each of the continuing education deficiencies. Said hours shall not count for continuing education renewal requirements for the next biennium.

Section Ten: Review and Practice Questions

Things You Should Probably Know
NOT Comprehensive

Class I Institutional Pharmacy
- Nursing home

Class II Institutional Pharmacy
- Hospital

Modified Class II Institutional Pharmacy
- Short-term or primary care treatment modalities in entities such as primary alcoholism treatment centers, free-standing emergency rooms, rapid in/out surgical centers, certain county health programs, and correctional institutions.
- Require a consultant pharmacist on record that must come on-site at least monthly
- Must have a protocol and policy and procedure manual
    - Type A – not more than 15 drugs on formulary and stored in bulk. Controlled substances allowed but <100 dosage units.
    - Type B – medications stored in patient specific form and bulk
    - Type C – medications stored in bulk and have an expanded formulary

Community pharmacy
- Independent or chain store
- May do parenteral/enteral or sterile compounding without obtaining an additional permit

Special-Limited Community Permit
- Obtained by a Class II institutional pharmacy to dispense medications to:
    - Employees, medical staff and dependents

- - Patients of the hospital not to exceed a 3 day supply
  - Emergency department patients

Special Non-Resident Pharmacy
- Mail order
- Pharmacy and pharmacist manager must be licensed in state of location
- Must be open at least 6 days and 40 hours per week
- Must have toll-free number

Special ALF
- For assisted living facilities providing medications
- Medications must be in patient specific unit dose packaging
- Consultant pharmacist required

Nuclear Pharmacy
- Traditional nuclear pharmacy
- Pharmacy technicians may accept oral prescriptions
- Nuclear pharmacist must always be present

What are the label requirements on a prescription?
- Name and address of the pharmacy.
- Date of dispensing.
- Serial number.
- Name of the patient or, if the patient is an animal, the name of the owner and the species of animal.
- Name of the prescriber.
- Name of the drug dispensed (except where the prescribing practitioner specifically requests that the name is to be withheld).
- Directions for use.
- Expiration date.
- If the medicinal drug is a controlled substance, a warning that it is a crime to transfer the drug to another person.

How long must most records be kept?
 2 years minimum

What is the minimum age to apply for a pharmacy permit?
> 18 years of age

Are pharmacies allowed to have referral arrangements with physicians or any other type of provider?
> No

Are pharmacists allowed to administer the flu vaccine?
> Yes if they have received the required training and are insured and under a protocol with a licensed physician.

What are the different sterile compounding risk levels?
> See sterile compounding definitions

What is the makeup of the Board of Pharmacy?
> 7 pharmacists and 2 Florida residents

How do you retire a pharmacist license? And reactivate it?
- Place the license on retired status – submit written request to the board and pay fee
- Reactivating a retired license – must have all the required CE from each biennium the license was retired and pay all fees
    - If inactive for less than 5 years – must pass the MPJE
    - If inactive for 5 or more years – must pass the NAPLEX and MPJE

How to reinstate a delinquent license?
- An active or inactive license that is not renewed by midnight of the expiration date of the license shall automatically revert to delinquent status
- Reinstate a pharmacist delinquent license = complete all CE requirements and pay fees
- Reinstate a delinquent consultant pharmacist license = pay fees

- Reinstate a delinquent nuclear pharmacist license = pay fees
- Reinstate a delinquent registered pharmacy technician = complete all CE requirements and pay fees
- A license in delinquent status that is not renewed prior to midnight of the expiration date of the current licensure cycle shall be rendered null and must apply for a new license

How many hours of CE are required for a pharmacist license and in what time frame?
- 30 hours in previous 24 months
- 2 hours on medication errors required
- First renewal must have 1 hour of HIV/AIDS
- At least 10 hours must be live

Consultant pharmacist CE requirements
- Minimum of 24 hours of CE required for license renewal in addition to the 30 hours required to renew a pharmacist license

Nuclear pharmacist CE requirements
- Minimum of 24 hours of CE required for license renewal in addition to the 30 hours required to renew a pharmacist license

Registered pharmacy technician CE requirements
- 20 hours of CE required prior to license renewal
- 1 hour of HIV/AIDS upon first renewal
- Minimum of 4 live hours

Pharmacist to intern ratio
- 1:1

How many intern hours are required for licensure by examination?

- 2080 hours

What is the minimum age to apply for a pharmacist license?
- 18 years of age

What are the responsibilities of a pharmacy technician?
- Registered pharmacy technicians may assist the pharmacist in performing the following tasks:
    - Retrieval of prescription files, patient files and profiles and other such records pertaining to the practice of pharmacy;
    - Data Entry;
    - Label preparation;
    - The counting, weighing, measuring, pouring and compounding of prescription medication or stock legend drugs and controlled substances, including the filling of an automated medication system;
    - Initiate communication to a prescribing practitioner or their medical staffs (or agents) regarding patient prescription refill authorization requests. For the purposes of this section "prescription refill" means the dispensing of medications pursuant to a prescriber's authorization provided on the original prescription;
    - Initiate communication to confirm the patient's name, medication, strength, quantity, directions and date of last refill;
    - Initiate communication to a prescribing practitioner or their medical staff (or agents) to obtain clarification on missing or illegible dates, prescriber name, brand/generic preference, quantity, DEA registration number or license numbers; and
    - May accept authorization for a prescription renewal. For the purposes of this section, "prescription renewal" means the dispensing of

medications pursuant to a practitioner's authorization to fill an existing prescription that has no refill remaining.
- Registered Pharmacy technicians shall not:
    - Receive new verbal prescriptions or any change in the medication, strength or directions;
    - Interpret a prescription or medication order for therapeutic acceptability and appropriateness;
    - Conduct a final verification of dosage and directions;
    - Engage in prospective drug review;
    - Provide patient counseling;
    - Monitor prescription usage; and
    - Override clinical alerts without first notifying the pharmacist.

What is the pharmacist to registered pharmacy technician ratio?
- 1:1 unless received special approval by the board.

How many hours of training for a nuclear pharmacist license?
- Minimum of 500 hours

What is the minimum age for a registered pharmacy technician license?
- 17 years of age

How long must CE records be kept?
- At least 2 years

Does an out of state pharmacy that mails prescriptions to Florida residents need to have a Florida pharmacy permit? Do the pharmacists need to be licensed in Florida?
- Yes, the Special – Nonresident pharmacy permit
- No the pharmacy manager needs to be licensed in their state of location.

What happens if a pharmacist fails to notify law enforcement in the required time frame after learning of any instance in which a person obtained or attempted to obtain a controlled substance through fraudulent methods?
- Considered to have committed a misdemeanor of the first degree

Pharmacist responsibilities
- Supervise and be responsible for the controlled substance inventory.
- Receive verbal prescriptions from a practitioner.
- Interpret and identify prescription contents.
- Engage in consultation with a practitioner regarding interpretation of the prescription and date in patient profile.
- Engage in professional communication with practitioners, nurses or other health professionals.
- Advise or consult with a patient, both as to the prescription and the patient profile record.
- When parenteral and bulk solutions of all sizes are prepared, regardless of the route of administration, the pharmacist must:
    o Interpret and identify all incoming orders.
    o Mix all extemporaneous compounding or be physically present and give direction to the registered pharmacy technician for reconstitution, for addition of additives, or for bulk compounding of the parenteral solution.
    o Physically examine, certify to the accuracy of the final preparation, thereby assuming responsibility for the final preparation.
    o Systemize all records and documentation of processing in such a manner that professional responsibility can be easily traced to a pharmacist.
- Only a pharmacist may make the final check of the completed prescription thereby assuming the complete responsibility for its preparation and accuracy.

Rules for a pharmacist's break
- May take a 30 minute break without the pharmacy closing
- Must have a sign present indicating hours of break and that the pharmacist is present
- Pharmacy technicians may release already checked prescriptions
- Must remain on the premises

Prescription refills
- Max of one year
- Six months for controlled substances and/or 5 refills
- No refills for C2s

Who can accept an oral prescription? Pharmacist? Registered pharmacy intern? Registered pharmach technician?
- Pharmacist and registered pharmacy intern only

Can pharmacists or pharmacies advertise medicinal drugs?
- Yes but not controlled substances

Who can transfer prescriptions? Pharmacist? Registered pharmacy intern? Registered pharmacy technician?
- Pharmacist and registered pharmacy intern only

What is the maximum days supply allowed to be dispensed by a pharmacist written prescription?
- 34 days or the standard treatment duration

Can pharmacists write for fluoride?
- Yes
- Cannot switch products
- Maximum duration of one year

A pharmacist can substitute a generically equivalent drug product for a brand name prescription drug except when?
- Prescriber must write the words "MEDICALLY NECESSARY" in his or her own handwriting on the face of the prescription if they want the brand name product

Which drugs are on the negative formulary?
- Digitoxin
- Conjugated Estrogen
- Dicumarol
- Chlorpromazine (Solid Oral Dosage Forms)
- Theophylline (Controlled Release)
- Pancrelipase (Oral Dosage Forms)

Rules for samples
- Unlawful to sell samples
- Pharmacies can only have samples of the drugs that may be ordered by a pharmacist
- Institutional pharmacies may possess sample medicinal drugs upon the written request of the prescribing practitioner.
- Those community pharmacies that are pharmacies of health care entities may possess sample medicinal drugs upon the written request of the prescribing practitioner.

Can pharmacies compound commercially available medications?
- Yes, the preparation of commercially available products from bulk when the prescribing practitioner has prescribed the compounded product on a per prescription basis and the patient has been made aware that the compounded product will be prepared by the pharmacist. The reconstitution of commercially available products pursuant to the manufacturer's guidelines is permissible without notice to the practitioner.

Are emergency refills allowed?

- Yes for a 72 hour supply max. If under a state of emergency then 30 days allowed.

How often must pharmacists renew their license?
- Every two years

What are the counseling requirements?
- A verbal and printed offer to counsel must be done with each new or refill prescription.

Which types of pharmacies must have a consultant pharmacist on record?
- Class I, a Class II, or a Modified Class II Institutional

How often must the consultant pharmacist inspect the facility?
- Monthly

Which form is used to destroy controlled substances?
- DEA form 41

How often is a pharmacy inspected by the board?
- At least once per year

What are the library requirements?
- A current pharmacy reference compendium such as the United States Pharmacopoeia/National Formulary, the U.S. Dispensatory, USP DI, (United States Pharmacopoeial Drug Information), the Remington Practice of Pharmacy, Facts and Comparisons or an equivalent thereof sufficient in scope to meet the professional practice needs of that pharmacy and a current copy of the laws and rules governing the practice of pharmacy in the State of Florida. If sterile compounding done then need Handbook of Injectable Drugs by American Society of Hospital Pharmacists. If a sterile compounding pharmacy then "Practice Guidelines For Personnel Dealing With Cytotoxic Drugs" is also required.

What is the beyond use date of a customized patient medication package?
- Not more than 60 days

How many hours must a pharmacy be open per week?
- At least 40 hours

If a community pharmacy is closed, may someone enter without a pharmacist present?
- No

How often must the prescription drug stock be examined for expired medications?
- At least every 4 months

Can a prescription drug be returned to stock if brought back by a patient?
- Only if it is in a closed drug delivery system in which unit dose or customized patient medication packages are dispensed to in-patients

When does the board need to be notified about a loss of data?
- Within 10 days

Can a central fill pharmacy deliver controlled substance prescriptions to a consumer?
- No

Some central fill pharmacy rules
- May deliver medications to the consumer if
    - Both pharmacies under same ownership or have a contract
    - Must have a pharmacist available at least 40 hours per week
    - Toll-free number for counseling

- o Each pharmacies name and address must be on the prescription label
- o No controlled substances
- May fax prescriptions to the central fill pharmacies
- Keep all records at least two years from date of last fill

Can prescribers at a hospital with a class II pharmacy permit dispense prescription drugs from the emergency department?
- Yes but a max of 24 hour supply and must follow labeling requirements for prescriptions.

How long records must be kept for pharmacist administration of influenza vaccines?
- Minimum 5 years

How many hours of training are required for pharmacists to administer the influenza vaccine?
- 20 hours

What are the requirements for writing multiple controlled substance prescriptions?
- Cannot have controlled substances from different classes on the same prescription blank
- A controlled substance cannot be on the same prescription blank as a medicinal drug (not a controlled substance)

Can a controlled substance prescription written by an out of state prescriber be filled at a Florida pharmacy?
- Yes but pharmacist must validate the identity of the prescriber if not known to them, must be issued pursuant to a valid patient-physician relationship, and that it is authentic and drugs or medicinal supplies so ordered are considered necessary for the continuation of treatment of a chronic or recurrent illness.

Can a prescriber call in a prescription for a controlled substance?
- Yes but maximum of 30-day supply of a Schedule III upon an oral prescription issued in this state

What are the controlled substance prescription label requirements?
- The name and address of the pharmacy from which such controlled substance was dispensed.
- The date on which the prescription for such controlled substance was filled.
- The number of such prescription, as recorded in the prescription files of the pharmacy in which it is filled.
- The name of the prescribing practitioner.
- The name of the patient for whom, or of the owner and species of the animal for which, the controlled substance is prescribed.
- The directions for the use of the controlled substance prescribed in the prescription.
- A clear, concise warning that it is a crime to transfer the controlled substance to any person other than the patient for whom prescribed.

Can schedule II prescriptions be called in by the prescriber?
- No except for an emergency refill

What is the maximum supply that can be dispensed for a schedule II emergency refill?
- 72 hour supply

Controlled substance prescription requirements
- For Schedule II-IV must have the quantity written out and numerically noted AND must have the abbreviated month written out on the prescription
- The full name and address of the person for whom, or the owner of the animal for which, the controlled substance is dispensed.

- The full name and address of the prescribing practitioner and the practitioner's federal controlled substance registry number shall be printed thereon.
- If the prescription is for an animal, the species of animal for which the controlled substance is prescribed.
- The name of the controlled substance prescribed and the strength, quantity, and directions for use thereof.
- The number of the prescription, as recorded in the prescription files of the pharmacy in which it is filled.
- The initials of the pharmacist filling the prescription and the date filled.

Does the person picking up a controlled substance prescription have to show identification?
- Yes the pharmacist must obtain suitable identification from the patient prior to dispensing a Schedule II-IV however exempt if dispensed by mail and the patient has insurance.

Can physician assistants and advanced nurse practitioners write for prescription medications?
- Yes they may prescribe drugs that are not controlled substances as long as they are under the supervision of a licensed practitioner.
- Must include the supervising practitioner's name and professional license number on the prescription and on the dispensed drug container.

What are the maximum amounts of pseudoephedrine someone can purchase?
- Max in a single day to an individual = 3.6 grams
- Max of 3 packages in any single, retail, over-the-counter sale
- Max in a 30 day period = 9 grams

Can an automatic pharmacy system used at a long term care facility or hospice, or a state correctional institution dispense controlled substances?
- Yes but a separate DEA registration from the provider pharmacy is required for each remote site

Review Questions

1. How many CE hours are required every 2 years for pharmacist license renewal
    a. 15
    b. 20
    c. 25
    d. 30

2. How many CE hours are required to be from live sources every 2 years for pharmacist license renewal
    a. 0
    b. 5
    c. 10
    d. 15

3. How many hours of CE are required to renew a consultant pharmacist license
    a. 12
    b. 24
    c. 30
    d. 35

4. How many hours of CE are required to renew a nuclear pharmacist license
    a. 12
    b. 24
    c. 30
    d. 35

5. How many CE hours are required for a registered pharmacy technician license renewal
    a. 5
    b. 10
    c. 20
    d. 30

6. How many CE hours are required to be obtained live for registered pharmacy technician license renewal
    a. 0
    b. 1
    c. 2
    d. 3
    e. 4

7. How many CE hours are required to be on medication errors for both pharmacists and technician license renewals
    a. 0
    b. 1
    c. 2
    d. 3

8. How many hours of training are required before pharmacists can administer immunizations
    a. 0
    b. 10
    c. 15
    d. 20

9. How old must someone be to apply for pharmacist by examination
    a. No minimum age
    b. 17
    c. 18
    d. 20

10. How long are examination scores good for when applying for licensure by examination
    a. 1 year
    b. 2 years
    c. 3 years
    d. Never expire

11. What is the required passing score on the foreign pharmacy graduate equivalency examination
    a. 70%
    b. 75%
    c. 80%
    d. 85%

12. How many internship hours are required to be completed for licensure
    a. 1500
    b. 1580
    c. 2080
    d. 2500

13. If a license has been retired for more than 5 years and the licensee wants it to be reinstated, what tests are required
    a. NAPLEX
    b. MJPE
    c. Both NAPLEX and MPJE
    d. No tests are required

14. If a license has been retired for less than 5 years and the licensee wants it to be reinstated, what tests are required
    a. NAPLEX
    b. MJPE
    c. Both NAPLEX and MPJE
    d. No tests are required

15. How many hours of supervised work activity in Florida are foreign graduates required to obtain
    a. 100
    b. 180
    c. 500
    d. 580

16. How many years of active practice must a pharmacist obtain inorder to apply for licensure by endorsement
    a. 1 year in the previous 5 years
    b. 1 year in the previous 7 years
    c. 2 years in the previous 5 years
    d. 2 years in the previous 7 years

17. How many members make up the Board of Pharmacy
    a. 6
    b. 7
    c. 8
    d. 9

18. Who/Whom appoints members of the Board of Pharmacy
    a. Voters
    b. Governor
    c. Senate
    d. House

19. How many members of the Board of Pharmacy must be licensed pharmacists
    a. 6
    b. 7
    c. 8
    d. 9

20. What is the minimum age to become a pharmacy technician
    a. 15
    b. 16
    c. 17
    d. 18

21. How many registered technicians may a pharmacist supervise without additional approval from the board
    a. 1

  b. 2
  c. 3
  d. Unlimited

22. With special approval from the board, what is the maximum number of registered pharmacy technicians a pharmacist may supervise
  a. 1
  b. 2
  c. 3
  d. Unlimited

23. An intern may begin employment as an intern in a Florida pharmacy while waiting to be registered by the Department of Health.
  a. True
  b. False

24. How many hours of formal didactic training are required for a pharmacist to become a licensed nuclear pharmacist
  a. 100
  b. 200
  c. 250
  d. 500

25. How many hours of on-the-job training in the handling of radiopharmaceuticals are required to be licensed as a nuclear pharmacist
  a. 100
  b. 200
  c. 250
  d. 500

26. What are the maximum amount of CE hours that can be counted per biennium by attending a Board of Pharmacy meeting
  a. 5

    b. 10
    c. 15
    d. 20

27. How many hours of training are required for a pharmacist to be certified to administered influenza vaccines
    a. 5
    b. 10
    c. 15
    d. 20

28. Interns may only perform acts relating to the filling, compounding, or dispensing of medicinal drugs unless it is done under the direct and immediate personal supervision of a person actively licensed to practice pharmacy in this state.
    a. True
    b. False

29. Who can accept an oral prescription
    a. Pharmacist
    b. Pharmacist intern under supervision of a pharmacist
    c. Pharmacy technician under supervision of a pharmacist
    d. All of the above
    e. A and B

30. A prescription for a non-controlled medication is only valid for
    a. 6 months
    b. 12 months
    c. 24 months
    d. No expiration date

31. Animal shelters have which type of pharmacy permit

a. Modified Class II Institutional Pharmacy Permit
b. Class I Pharmacy Permit
c. Class II Pharmacy Permit
d. Special Pharmacy Permit

32. A mail service pharmacy located in another state must notify the Florida Board of Pharmacy when there is a change in
    a. Prescription department managers
    b. Location
    c. Corporate officers
    d. A and C
    e. All of the above

33. Pharmacies may advertise the sale of controlled substances.
    a. True
    b. False

34. Pharmacists may dispense a one-time emergency refill.
    a. True
    b. False

35. What is the maximum amount that may be dispensed in an one-time emergency refill
    a. 24 hour supply
    b. 48 hour supply
    c. 72 hour supply
    d. 96 hour supply

Answers

1. D – 30
2. C – 10
3. B – 24
4. B – 24
5. C – 20
6. E – 4
7. C – 2
8. D – 20
9. C – 18
10. C – 3 years
11. B – 75%
12. C – 2080
13. C – Both NAPLEX and MPJE
14. B – MPJE
15. C – 500
16. C – 2 years in previous 5 years
17. D – 9
18. B – Governor
19. B – 7
20. C – 17
21. A – 1
22. C – 3
23. B – False
24. B – 200
25. D – 500
26. B – 10
27. D – 20
28. A – True
29. E – A and B
30. B – 12 months
31. A – Modified Class II Institutional Pharmacy Permit
32. E – All of the above
33. B – False
34. A – True

35. C – 72 hour supply

Made in the USA
Middletown, DE
06 June 2015